THERAPEUTIC TANTRA

THERAPEUTIC TANTRA

THE POWER OF PHYSICAL, PSYCHOLOGICAL AND SPIRITUAL HEALING

SADHU SANTIDEVA

COSMO PUBLICATIONS
2025 New Delhi

THERAPEUTIC TANTRA.
THE POWER OF PHYSICAL
PSYCHOLOGICAL AND SPIRITUAL HEALING

First Published 2001
SECOND IN PRINT 2025

ISBN 81-7755-159-0

Published by
COSMO PUBLICATIONS
for
GENESIS PUBLISHING PVT. LTD.
24-B, Ansari Road, Darya Ganj,
New Delhi-110 002,
INDIA

Printed in India

CHAPTER-1

SALIENT FEATURES OF TANTRA

CHAPTER - 1

A. What is Tantra:

Desire of pleasure and removal of pain was and still is the human tendency. Like other communities of the world, Hindus also believed that they were surrounded by supernatural powers which they considered as the cause of their pleasure and pain. For the benign influence of power and removal of the evil impact, they gave them a status of deity and worshipped them through Mantras. The important occasions which start from the conception of womb to the cremation ground, according to the oriental view, they are sixteen in number, known as Sodàs Samskàras, the human subject is protected from the evil influences through the proounciation of Mantras as a part of certain ritualistic pattern of tradition.

Physical disorders and mental ailments also were considered as wrath of supernatural power. For this they have worked out Mantric therapy, in which Màntra is considered as having healing power. Does Mantra really contain such power ? Apparently it looks as a collection of syllabus but in reality they are highly potent but their prtency is latent. One has to charge the Mantra with his own inner power for the desired results. But how to charge ? Or how to awaken the inner latent power ? As we have seen both in the preface and in the introduction that Tantra shows the way of expansion of inner power . But what Tantra is ? One may have question . This chapter is chiefly devoted for the exposition of the Subtle and sound meaning of Tantra and its related notions.

Lexical and esoteric meaning of Tantra:

Many definitions have been give for the term 'Tantra'. In the Samskrit lexicon the term Tantra has used in many senses. This term is derived from the rootütan means 'to spread out'.[1] But what is to be spread out? It is the spreading out the expansion of worldly and other worldly knowledge.[2] Esoterically, the meaning expansion also represents the cultivation of latent physical and mental powers.

Now let us penetrate deeper into the very term and see what it represents ? The term Tantra is a combination of two world namely, Tanoti and Tràyate which stand for expansion and liberation respectively. But what is to be expanded and what is to be liberated ? Here it is an expansion of mind and liberation of energy. Let us illustrate this point.

Mind functions within a specific circle or limit. It work through the date give by senses. We can see only those thgings which our optic system allows us to see. We can not see behind the wall with naked eyes. There are also minute objects in the world which we can not see through eyes because of its limitations. Like wise, we can hear only those voices which come from the specific range. Same is the case with all senses. This indicates that mind is dependent on sense stimuli and because of this its experiences are very limited.

If we break the boundaries of mind, it can have infinite experiences of varied types. Just now it is a slave of senses. If it comes out of the clutches of sense organs, it can flow every where and can enjoy desired experiences. This can happen only after the expansion or liberation of mind from the clutches of sense organs. Simultaneously, the modification of the powers of sense or the transformation of senses through certain practice also expands the area of the functions of mind infinitely.

How Tantra help in this regards ? Tantra sheds light on the way of expansion though techniques (One of the meaning of Tantra is also technique). Tantra says that allow your mind to move every where. Expand the area of mind.[3] Mantra helps in this regards. It's a vehicle for awakening the deeper forces lying within one self. A sound is a wave which carries electrical vibration of energy. The pronounciation of Mantra gives a new dimension to consciousness which penetrates deeper into inner recesses of mind.

For this, Tantra has also prescribed unique types of method of meditation. Tantra is also meditation, but it is a meditation though symbols. These may be linguistic syllables (Mantra) or geographical figures (Yantra). Tantric way of dealing with mind is that, in which one has to attend each and every thought as a mere witness or seer and not to suppress the thought Give total independence one can come out from the boundaries of mind and can expand the arena of mind because only unconditioned mind and can realise the infinite. The observations of Dr. Lalan Prasad also leads us to this fact. In his own words, "Tantra Sàdhanà therefore means a spiritual path which leads to the expansion of one's mental objectivity. Meanxs "the arena of mental projection is also increased. When a Sàdhaka attains the projection of mental arena of 360^0, he becomes one with the cosmic mind".[4]

This is about the former portion of the term Tantra, that is Tanyate. Now something about the later portion of the term, that is Trayate. As we have seen, Tràyate stands for the meaning "liberation". We can liberate only those things which are in bondage. For Tàntra, Kundalinì, the cosmic universal energy, lying dormant in human body in the pelvic region or the Mùlàdharà cakra in coiled form is to be liberated. If once the Sadhaka (practitioner) liberates this energy, he becomes the master of all manifestations of energy because he has gripped the very source of energy. The way of liberation is the very core of Tantra Sàdhanà.

The other meaning of Tantra is that which saves or protects.[5] It saves the Sàdhaka from the wordly bondage by the constant meditation (Manana) of the Highest Reality in the form of Mantra.[6] It also protects Sadhaka from physical and mental ailments. Thus it works as a Therapy. The Sàbdakai padrum, a Samskrit dictionary also gives the meaning of the term Tantra in which it declares Tantra as medicine and doctrine.[7]

So Tantra saves Sadhaka both as knowledge and as therapy. With the lamp of knowledge it saves Sadhaka from the darkness of nescience and with the healing process it protects him from physical and mental disorders. Hence it saves Sadhaka from both, spiritual as well as psycho-somatic calamities. It is rightly remarked by Hastings in the encyclopedia of Religion and Ethics That, it has been estimated that two-thirds of Hindu religions and one-third of Hindu medicine is Tantric.[8]

In the meanings of Tantra, give by the Sabdakalpadruma, we

have seen that, term tantra also signifies the doctrine or system, (Siddhanta). So any philosophy can be called Tantra. For instance, Samkhya tantra, Gautamiya Tantra etc. The great vedantist Sree Samkaracharya has also used the term "Vainasika Tantra" for the ksanabhangavada of the Buddhists.[9]

The term Àgama is the synonyme of Tantra.[10] The definition give by the Param Samhita, a Vaisnava Tantra includes all Siva, Sakti and Visnu aspects. According to it, Àgama is that which comes from Siva goes to Parvati and is approved by Vasudeva.[11]

With the help of such information, without having any hesitation, we can say that Tantra is not a cheap literature of ghost and globin or a cult of black magic and sorceries as it is so considered. Tantra is a process or method which leads Sàdhaka to the self-realization though the cultivation of inner forces. Here we close this point with the mystic definition of Tantra given by Dr. Lalan Prasad Singh. "The mystic definition of Tantra is that it is a spiritual cult which liberates from the bondage of crudenessand ignorance. The word ta is the bija-Mantra (acoustic root) or crudness. Tantra is a process of Sàdhana which relieves one from the fetters of crudeness (ta). Thus , Tantra is an intuitional science which stands for the progressive realization of the Divine. It liberates one from the cimmerian darkness and leads into the divine effulgence. It is a path of Salvation. It is a science of the soul. The authoritative definition of the Tantra, is that which brings emancipation from the bondage of Màyà (tatra ya ayat tràyet yastu sa tantra parikìrtitah)."[12]

After having been acquainted with the meaning of Tantra one may be eager to know about its antiquity or tradition. Now let us glance over its tradition.

B. Tàntric Tradition:

Indian spiritual heritage is contained in scriptures. Various scriptures show us different ways which culminate at one point. Tantra is also one of them. It is the greatest path which has been forgotten rather neglected. The saviour of Tantra Arthur Avalon has tried to give a vivid description of supremacy of Tantra. Let us have a pleasure in his own words, "In this great festival, in this ancient Durgà festival of India, astrology, philosophy, smriti, purana, Veda, Vedànta and many other musical instruments are playing in the extensive court-yard of the universe. But we are grieved to find that the great instruments of the Tantra Sàstra, in which all other instrument are included, on which all other instruments depend, and which is the sole source of al Yantras and Mantras, is today silent"[13]. This is not a fancy but it secures sound base which is also reflected in the view of Dasgupta, S.B. who concludes all the esoteric schools as the off-shoots of Tantricism.[14] Off-shoot pre-supposes seed which is under the soil. But the question is : when the Tantra seed had been planted ? For this let us proceed with the Tantra antiquity.

Antiquity of Tantra is a very controversial problem. A complete and decided answer to this enigma has not yet been given. Antiquity can be answered only in terms of time but not in terms of soundness of principles. Ancientness is not the only measurement for the justification of any system but it should have some sound base. Tàntric tradition is fortunate to have both ancientness and soundness. For ancientness we will have to go back Indus-Valley civilization. (3500 B.C).

There is a great controversy among the scholar whether Tantra has its origin in Veda or vice versa. The reports of the excavations of Indus-Valley civilization, before the Aryan came into India, have favoured the first possibility.

Siva and Sakti symbols are highly attached with the Tàntric metaphysics. They were so deeply rooted in the mind of pre-Aryan people that they took the form of Gramdevatà. The idol of Siva and Sakti was and still being worshipped by each and every village. We shall expound this view with the help of the authentic report of the archaeologist Donald Mackenzie. As he reports, "The clay figures and images and phallic bactylic stones suggest that `Durga' and `Siva' worship was of a much greater antiquity in India than has hitherto been supposed.[15] Ghose, N.N. also supports the same view. "..people wee also intensely religious is proved by the discovery of a number of beautiful temples still preserved in fine shape, which they used as places of worship of the Mother Goddess and three headed Siva."[16]

Vedas are composed by the Àryan people while Tantra is the gift of pre-Àryan civilization. Dr. Lalan Prasad emphatically declares that, "From al these available historical evidence, it can be said with certainty that Tantra is the cult and spiritual faith of ancient India. It is the gift of the non-Àryan civilization."[17] The view of the Ram Chandra Rao is nothing but the echo of the above mentioned views. The origins are lost in the pre-history. In any case is is as old as Veda may be older.[18] Here Ram Cahndra Rao accepts the ancientness of Tantra than Veda as possibility. But he is sure to accept Tantra as old as Veda. As we know in Veda, we found ample references of Siva-Sakti which are the Tantric deities. The Rgveda and the Atharvaveda also contain many Suktas, like Ratri Sukta, Prithvi Sukta, Usa Sukta etc. and also Purusa Sukta, Rudra Sukta, which are related with female and male deities. This is enough pointer to declare Tantra as much older than Veda. Here the view of Nandulal Kundu will not be out of place. In his own worlds. "It is remarkable fact to be noted here that no where in some of the oldest Tantras such as the 'Màlini-Vijaya Tantra' the Rudra-Yàmala Tantra etc., no trace of the vedic influence and no mention of the vedas can be found; whereas in the Vedas we have clear evidence of Tàntric influence or influence of the `Àgama' and `Nigama' which go to prove that before the Àryans migrated to the Indian soil, the Tantras and Tàntric Cult were there as forming the core of the non-Aryan or the pre-Aryan civilization."[19]

Saivism and Sàktism are the schools of the Tantra-tradition. Both Siva and Sakti as god and goddess were prevalent in the non-Àryan Cult. We again here quote Ghose, N.N. regarding this. "The religion of the people seems to be iconic, the image of Siva taking the place of honour. The worship of phallic emblems, the linga and the yoni also prevalid.[20] This necessarily leads us to conclude that Saivism and Sàktism are the two pillars on which the spiritual edifice of non-Àryan was established.

Here we have tried to prove Tantra as much older than Veda

in terms of time. But this does not mean that they are contrary to each other. In the Tantric treatise like the 'Kulàrnava' and the 'Mahànirvàna' Tantra it is declared that Tantra is a scripture for the kaliyuga while Veda is for the Satyayuga[21] The one principle is presented in different ways according to the moral standard of the people of the particular age. We are the people having limited life-span and senses. It is impossible to grasp Vedas that is why Lord siva has gifted Tantra for the people of the Kaliyuga, Arthur Avalon has beautifully compromised this controversy by declaring Tantra as a perfume existing in Vedic Flower.[22] It can be further asked who has perfumed the Vedic flower ? For this, let us proceed towards the founder of Tantra.

C. Founders of Tantra

Vedic Flower is perfumed by Tantra. But who has perfumed Tantra is our problem of investigation. Though we know very little about it. Scholars have tried to fix the authorship of Tantra. There are two superficial contrary views regarding this nation among them one supports divien origin while the other favours human authorship, whoever may secure the authorship, we are not concerned with it. We are highly concerned with the core of philosophy. Any system can endure only by the strength of its essence. We have seen that Tantric philosophy has been prevalent since five thousand years if not more. This is enough evidence of its soundness. This soundness is infused by divine forces. How is it so ? For this we will have to peep into the related notions of this concept.

Tantra is generally considered as Àgama. Each syllable of this term is Full of significance. As Chakravarti, C., notes. "The term Àgama is explained as that class of Tantra which is addressed to Parvati by Siva.[23]" This exposition supports divine origin. But at the same time we have got some other Tantras which are associated with human names. For instance, Sanat Kumàra, Dattàtreya etc. Who are considered as authors of several Tanras. Of course, they were not lay man like us but at the same time we cannot consider them as Lord Siva. We have accepted them only as seers.

Dr. Lalan Prasad has very distinctly worked out the authorship.

He is against accepting all these scriptures as of divine origin. In his own words, "But from our point of view neither Tantra nor the Vedas are of divine origin. Both embody the intuitive vision of seers. The god head of the Vedas and of Tantra is an infinite, eternal, formless and transcendental entity. It is not a personal god. It does not have any vocal chord. There is no transcendental validity in the argument that Tantra or Veda is the voice of providence (Àpta Vàkya)."[24] Not with standing, he accepts Siva as originator of Tàntra but not Siva as we have accepted as god. In his own words, "The Founder of Tantra is Lord Siva. He is known as Àdi Guru. He is a great ascetic (Mahà yogi) and a great Tàntrika (Mahà kaula) he has oneness with the supreme God. He attained occult powers through Tantra Sadhana. It is beyond human mind to measure the depth and dimension of his spiritual power and personality. People revered, worshipped and adored him in ancient times. He is conceived to be Gunàtità and Nirguna Purusa.[25]

The great adherant of Tantra, Arthur Avalon differs on this point. It seems that he has accepted the founders of Tantra not as a scholar but as a devotee. He has tried to prove conclusively that Vedas and Tantras are Apta Vàkya or voice of providence. As he thinks, "As the courtiers of a royal court are not the authors, but merely the interpreters of state crafts, so the truth seeing Risis are not the originators of the Sàdhana Sàstra, but rememberencers merely. It is not a Sàstra marred by mistake, errors and deception, Bhavan, the creator of all creatures, knower of all hearts, is its revealar.[26]

The above mentioned two points are opposed to each other but what I think is that, this controversy is only at an apparent levf. If we go into the root of these views we find that the both respected scholars represent their views from the same ground, that is the ground of consciousness. Let us diffuse this statement.

There is incredible movement in the universe in every atom. Movement is a characteristic of consciousness. Universe is a combination of different atoms and they are full of consciousness. Hence universe is nothing but the ocean of consciousness. The one and the same consciousness pervades in the man and in the animal world also. But what makes man superior to animal ? There are certain obstructions of nescience on consciousness. Only man possesses the capacity to remove these obstructions which is not possible for animal. Animal is at sub-consciousnes level while man is at self-conscious level. Beyond self-consciousness there are certain layers which are known as Super-consciousness. It is not easy to reach as it seems so. Man should have tremendous power to control the natural forces, then he can realize the identity with super-consciousness. Here individual self merges into universal self. At this level he secures all the powers which we ascribe to god. It is my humble view that Dr. Lalan Prasad thinks Siva as a founder of Tantra, as a realized soul or as a soul of super consciousness. Though consciousness is same in man and superman but he has shattered off all the limitations of name and form. This type of soul can not be earthly but a divine one as Arthur Avalon accepts. We can conclusively declare that both have accepted divine origin directly or indirectly. Voice of realised soul comes, from the domain of divinity and far remote from human territory.

What is that in the Tàntric perfume-which has fragranced all the scriptures ? It is not its hoary antiquity or divine authorship but its sound principles on which edifice of Tantra system stands. Now we shall try to see the bricks of Tantra edifice under the title "Principles of Tantra".

D. Principles of Tantra:

The solidity of edifice depends upon the firmness of foundation and quality of bricks. Tàntra principles are very sound on which Tantric system is still sustained since five thousand years.

1. *Principle of Polarity:*

The principle of polarity is the foundation stone of Tantra system. Before going into the root of this principle let us be acquainted with what polarity is. The term 'polarity' is related with the word 'pole'. The lexical meaning of the word 'pole' is either of the two points of a body in which the attractive or repulsive energy is concentrated, as e.g. in a magnet.[27]

Tàntra has very uniquely worked out these two poles in the human body which is symbolically represented in Tantric treatise as Siva-Sakti. Biologically, it represents the male-female poles which is pre-requisite for any creation.

Tàntric principle of polarity works not only at physical level but it also applies at universal level. For Tantra, like human, universe is also an off-spring of the Highest Reality. The literal meaning (Vàcyàrtha) of the First verse of the Saundraya laharì reflect this fact.[28] The same view is also depicted by the Rasàrnava Tantra in which siva tells Pravati that He is the Father and She is the Mother of the universe and worldly objects.[29]

2. Principle of Identity:

How this polarity resides in the human body ? Every human being contains these two poles within; one is expressed while the other is latent. The externally himself expressed pole indicates either male or female character. If a person is male, female is already there but in a latent form. Same is the case of female. This new concept in biology is known as b-sexuality. But is not a new notion for a Tàntric seer. It has already been revealed by them and expressed it in terms of Hermo-phrodite (Ardhànarìsvara). Let us see how the exponent of Tantra tradition, Ajit Mookerji throws light on this point. "The bi-sexual potential exist in equal male-female (M/F) ratio in the reproduction of prooy plasm. Visually it has been depicted as the form of Ardhanarisvara (Siva-Parvati), male and female attributes shown as part of the same body, hermophroditically joined. The idea that mascularity and feminity are tow factors is as illusory as that of the duality of body and soul.[30]

Siva and Sakti are the two poles of one thing. Tantra represents polarity but not duality. Siva and Sakti are not two ultimate Realities but they are identical. This identity has been profusely described in many Tantras. We here quote only one or two. In the Mahànirvàna Tantra Lord Siva emphatically tells Pàrvati that there is no difference between them.[31] The Suddha Siddhanta Paddhati of Goraksanàtha depicts the same truth by giving the illustration of moon and moon light. As moon light is not different from moon and moon can not exist without moonlight in the same way Siva and Sakti are identical.[32]

This identity is also explained with the help of the illustration of creation. In the process of creation Siva is not able to do anything without Sakti. Siva is considered as corpse (Sava) devoid of Sakti (i). The very first verse of the Saundraya Laharì purports the same view. In which it is declared that without the union of Siva-Sakti no creation is possible. Not only that but when Siva unites with Sakti only then he usable to do anything.[33] The Today Tantra also reflect the same view.[34] We can't go ahead without quoting the words of Sree Ràmakrisna which are cited by Swami Prabhavananda. "Shri Ràmkrisna was wont to say that just as fire and its burning power are inseparable, so inseparable are Brahma and Sakti". When I meditate upon Reality as at rest, he once remarked, "that is, without the activities of creation, preservation and dissolution. I call it Brahman. When I meditate upon Reality as creative, I call it Sakti. In either case I am concerned with one and the same truth, the difference being only in the name and aspect.[35]

3. *Macrocosm and Microcosm:*

Hence Siva and Sakti become the invisible seed of the full grown up tree of universe. As the seed pervades in the branches, in the fruits of the tree likewise, Siva and Sakti also pervade in the universe and in the human body also. This is enough to raise a question about the relationship between the universe (Macrocosm) and the individual self (Microcosm). If there is a cold in the universe, we also feel coldness. If there is a heat, we also feel heat in the body. How is it possible ? Tantra has found out that whatever is in universe also resides in human body. The third chapter of the Siddha-Siddhànta paddhati of Goràkanath is completely devoted to this aspect. The slighest change in universe consequently reflects in body. Thus Tantra accepts the identity between macrocosm and microcosm on which the whole astrology is based.

Being a replica of universe, body contains all whatever there is in the universe. Hence for the realization of Reality behind the universe, it is not necessary to roam into the world. Body is the best means for realization. The citation of the Ratnasara Tantra which is quoted by Ajit Mookerji is very suggestive. "He who realizes the truth of the body can then come to know the truth of the universe."[36]

4. *Concrete and positive view of Reality:*

This also reflects the view of Tantra about the nature of Reality. For Tantra, Reality is not an abstract entity but can be realized through physical or mortal body. Body is not merely a gross product of Prakriti but is a divine gift of nature and because of this, the Tantra like Kularnava declares body as the temple of God.[37] This reflects the positive view of Tantra regarding body element which is highly neglected by Jainism, Christianity and Buddhism.

This shows how human being enjoys great significance in Tantra tradition. The Kulàrnava Tantra has laid greater stress on this aspect. As Vishvasàra Tantra declares, "There is no birth like unto the human birth. Both Devas and pitras desire it. For the Jiva, the human body is out of all bodies, the most difficult to come by. For this, it is said that human birth is attained with extreme difficulty".[38]

Indian philosophy believes that soul has to cross the cycle of births according to the deeds he has committed in previous life. Human birth is the only birth in which he gets complete sway over the birth cycle by doing selfless deeds. (Niskàma karma). To do anything with or without intension is a property of mind. Hence mind should be first controlled. It is not the worldly objects that bind us but the attitudes of mind toward it creates pleasure and pain. This is the wisdom and ignorance of this is the knot of nescience. The knot should be broken and that is the liberation (Moksa) advocated by Tantra.[39]

But how mind becomes the cause of pleasure and pain ? It is the mental disposition (Bhàva) which is responsible for this and for Tantra mental disposition is the property of mind.[40] Worldly objects are neither good nor bad. They are as it is. But is our mental disposition towards them which binds us or liberates. Scriptures like Dharma Sàstra discloses this truth by giving illustration of a person who kisses his wife and his daughter with the same limb but with different intention.[41] So it is the mental outlook which distorts the world and not anything else. This fact is beautifully depicted by the Kaulàvali Tantra which is cited in the Karpura Stava Ràja.[42]

So mind can be the means for both bondage as well as Salvatio. Among all the mental instincts, sex is generally considered as the most binding and powerful one. But Tantra has a healthy view regarding this. Tantra views sex as a positive force. There are two possibilities in the utilization of this force. If it is misused, it may prove to be a curse and a source of misery. At the same time if it is used properly with understanding it proves to be boon. To utilize it as a boon or curse depends upon us. Tantra accepts the positivity of sex energy to that extent that it becomes the source of Salvation. Tantra shows the way of sublimation of that instinct which is generally considered as the cause of downfall.[43]

In conclusion we say that Tantra lays greater stress on mental aspect. As it is declared in the Kulàrnava Tantra, if anything is done with the purity of mind even sin becomes virtue and phenomenal world becomes door to divinity.[44] It would be more proper to say that the approach of Tantra is to avoid the two extremes, that is renunciation and indulgence. Thus it shows the balanced and healthy view regarding world and its affairs.

From this we can conclude without having hesitation that the bricks of Tantra edifice are very sound and rational. But what is that which has distort or Shaken the foundation of the system of Tantra ?

It is nothing but misinterpretation of its symbolic language which is responsible for this. One may wish to know which are the symbols and how they are unduely justified. For this let us see some of the Tantric Symbols with their proper significance with the help of Tantra treatise.

E10

It is a fact that the revealer of the epic Ramayana, the Valmiki was robber in his youth. One Vulnerable incident happened which changed a robber into risi. Which was that ? At one night some sages gave him a Mantra Ràma, a word symbol of the Higher Reality, for the repetition or japa. Constant repetition and concentration on the Mantra Ràma changed the entire personality of Valmiki. An ordinary man Valio transformed into sage Vàlmikì. What is that symbol one may wish to know.

From the instance of Vàlmiki, we could see that symbol is a medium through which one conveys his sentiments. He worshipped the Higher Reality through the word symbol Ràma. This medium can either be a language, figure or image. At initial level symbols are required for layman but not for the sàdhaka like Sree Ràmakrsna Paramhamsa, for whom everywhere there is a linga. He feels god not at particular place or in object but everywhere. This identity is the base of Indian symbolism. As Danielou, Alain observes, "The whole Hindu iconography is built on a code of symbols based on the assumption that there exists a natural affinity between forms and ideas.[45]

Tantra symbology is based on such a fact. All the natural forces are symbolized in a geometrical figures or in a language form which in Tantra terminology known as Yàntra and Mantra respectively. Details of Tàntric and Mantric symbology we shall see at proper place. Apart from Mantra and Yantras there are also some figures or symbols which have played prominent role in Tàntric symbolism. Here we shall try to see some of the Tàntric Symbols.

1. *Tantra Symbols:*

Tantra has been largely misunderstood for its symbolic language. The cause behind this is that, it represents subtle thought process of evolution and dissolution of universe in naked form without bringing any religion, social or political prejudices to bear upon. It's aim is out and spiritual which lifts man from his slumber to make him aware of the infinite potentialities with which he is endowed.

Now what Tantra believes regarding symbolism ? Like other systems, Tantra has considered two aspects of Reality. One is formless (Nirguna) while the other is with form (Saguna). As the Devi

Bhagavata declares, the formless Reality can not and will not be ever seen in the universe. All the perceived things are the combination of three reals of Reality, that is, Sattva, Rajas and Tamas. Hence each and every object of the world represents or is a symbolic presentation of the Higher Reality.[46] The Kulàrnava Tantra has beautifully expressed the importance of symbol. For its explanation it gives simply of cow. As milk of cow pervades in the whole body of cow but it comes only through udder like wise the all pervading formless Reality expresses itself through symbols. Worship of the particular symbol with full faith and devotion secures the attainment of the Reality.[47]

But how the all pervading deity is symbolized ? Tantra has symbolized it in a copulation form that is the union of Siva-Sakti or liñga-yoni. In the previous paragraph we have seen that Tantra has viewed energy as Mother, the female pole. But as we know, for any creation copulation with opposite pole is required. Hence Tantra has accepted male pole, which is known as Siva. This is not the duality but the polarity which is the pre-requirement for any creation. It seem that to avoid dualism and to project monism Tantra has utilized copulation symbol to represent the real nature of the Higher Reality. Here it is necessary to be clear that whenever Tantra has used the sexual symbology of Siva-Sakti, it has always viewed the union of positive and the negative aspect of Reality and not the physical copulation of gross linga and yoni it is generally considered. Sex in Tantra, is not a goal but the source of salvation. It is a path of love and not of lust. Now let us deal in detail the Tantra symbols with the help of Tantra texts. We shall start with the Symbol linga.

(a) Linga:

The most misunderstood Symbol, in Tantra Symbols is liñga. It is neglected only by considering it as mere phallus, the male generative organ. Why is it neglected ? The reason of it, is that, linga is related with the sex concepts and we consider sex as something obnoxious. Though we hate it apparently, we have accepted it internally but we feel inferiority to accept it. Tantra seers were very courageous in this regards. They have accepted sex positively. Not only that butalso gave a high status as a source of salvation.

We have see before that Tàntric view is out and out spiritual. It also views liñga in a spiritual manner. The Tantric text "Anubhava Sùtram" clearly declares the liñga as a source of creation and dissolution, that source is nothing but the Lord Siva Himself.[48] The another Tàntric text, the Vàtulsuddhàkhya Tantra also emphatically declares liñga as a creator and destroyer.[49]

This view is also supported by the Abhinava Gupta. In his Tantrà-loka, he declares that the wise man should consider liñga as a cause of creation and destruction. In the term linga, 'La' indicates dissolution (Laya) while 'Ga' stands for arrival (Àgamana). One should worship the Àtmalinga and avoid other lingas.[50] Not only above mentioned Tantras but puràna like Siva purana and liñga puràna also support the same view.

The Siva purana consider liñga as a first cause, the source of consciousness and substance of universe.[51] While according to the linga puràna, liàga is both the cause of dissolution and evolution.[52]

There are ample references in Tantra which suggest this meaning. The above mentioned references are enough to conclude that Tantra has not applied liñga as physical or gross phallus but as a prime cause of creation of universe. This view is also supported by Danielou, Alain, "When Hindus Worship the liñga, they do not deify a physical feature, they merely recognize the divine, eternal form manifest in the microcosm. It is the human phallus which is a divine emblem of the eternal causal form, the al pervading linga.[53]

A devotee worships linga. Like other forms of worship, this also secures some results. In other systems of Sàdhanà, Sàdhaka gains salvation through penance while Tàntric worship of linga is very positive in nature as it secures both indulgence and liberation. This uniqueness lies in the approach of Tantra towards sex. How it secures both that has been reflected in the view of karapàtriji, "Those who do not recognize the divine nature of the phallus, who do not measure the importance of sex ritual, who consider the act of love as low or contempatible or as a mere physical function, are bound to fail in their attempts at physical as well as spiritual achievement. To ignore the sacredness of the linga is dangerous, whereas through its worship the joy of life (bhukti) and the joy of liberation (Mukti) are obtained.[54]

Having seen something about the liñga concept let us proceed with the other symbol which is also related with sex notion, that is, symbol Harmophrodite. (Ardhanàrisvara).

(b) Ardhanàrìsvara:

We have been discussing about symbolism. Our first symbol was liñga in which we have considered linga as a source of creation. But as we know, only liñga or male pole is not sufficient for any creation. Creation is a result of copulation which demands on the other pole, that is yoni, the female pole. Tantra represents the Synthesized form of liñga-yoni or Siva-Sakti through the symbol of Ardhanàrìsvara or half male-half female form.

The concept of Ardhanarisvara is not a fancy of Tantra seers but it also contains both spiritual and scientific significance. Universe is a creation. This pre-supposes its creator who contains both positive and negative or M/F poles. Tantra has projected this polarity in the Higher Reality. The Tantric treatise the Saundrya Lahari very emphatically and beautifully declares universe as an off-spring of the universal parents the Siva-Sakti.[55] Tantra symbolizes these two inseparable and identical aspects of the Higher Reality in the form of Ardhanàrisvara. The Vital Suddhakhya Tantra also affirms this fact. As it declares linga is Siva and yoni is Sakti. Their copulation is the result into universe.[56]

Not only Tantras but Vedas also have mentioned the different pairs for pre-creation. A list of the pairs have been mentioned by Aggarwal, Vàsudeva, in his book "Siva Mahadeva".

But what these pairs indicate ? According to Tantra, these pairs of opposite is nothing but the form of energy. We may coin any name like Nara-Nàri, Kumàra-kumari, Siva-Pàrvati etc. but al these can he reduced into one Higher Reality, that is, for Tantra, is energy. When the creative positive energy combines with the negative energy, interaction starts which results into creation. Zimmer, Henrich views this fact like this: "As the symbol of male creative energy, the lingam is frequently combined with the primary symbol of female creative energy, the yoni, the later forming the base of the image with the former rising from its centre. This serves as a representation of the creative union that procreates and sustains the life of the universe. Liñgam and Yoni, Siva and his goddess, symbolize the antagonistic yet co-operative forces of the sexes. Their sacred Marriage (Greek : hieroes—gamos) is multifariously figured in the various traditions of world mytho-dlogy. They are the archetypal parents, Father and Mother of the world, themselves the first born of the pairs of opposites, first bifurcation of the primal cosmogenic reality, now re-united in productive harmony. Under the form of Father Heaven and Mother Earth they were known to the Greeks as Zeus and Hera, Uranos and Gaia, to the Chinese T'ien and Ti, Yang and Yin."[57]

Tantra projects the nature of Hermophrodite of Higher Reality in its manifestation, that is the objects of universe also. Being a part and parcel of the Higher Reality we also contain the same quality. Every male has female pole and female has male pole, in latent form. This Tantric truth has emerged out under the name of bi-sexuality in modern bio-physics. According to the law of bi-sexuality to tell somebody as mere male or female is opposed to the concept of bi-sexuality. We bifurcate the two sexes by the expressed pole. But in reality we are both male and female, Siva and Sakti.

Tantra is not only confined to the bi-sexuality but it has also located the exact place of male-female pole in the body where the bio-physics has yet to reach. According to the Tantra, the right side always represents male-sun or positive pole while the left side represents female moon or negative pole. In the Tripura Samhità. Devi declares, "The wise should know the basic fact that the female gene resides in the left side of all males. He can not discover the self when he is alienated from his own nature."[58]

Like liñga symbol, this has also been neglected on the ground that it is related with the sex drive. Tantra views sex as a means for realizing wholeness. Though we are infinite and whole, due to the lack of wisdom of it we constantly feel finiteness. That is why we always try to reach that wholeness. This fact is reflected by the attraction of the opposite sex. Man tries to fell completeness by uniting with the outer woman. Likewise Woman also feels wholeness by the unification with outer man. Tantra says that satisfaction of sex drive is the only easiest way for realizing infinite because it is our nature. Suppression of it will create nothing but disorders and distortion. In the words of Mookerji, Ajit, "The composite figure of Siva and Parvati as half male and half female indicates that male and female elements are balanced in both of them. Full emancipation is dependent upon our realization of this fact.[59]

In conclusion we can say without having any doubt that the symbol of Ardhanarivara has nothing to do with gross physical form of sex. On the contrary, it leads us from gross to subtle. As Sree Majithia views this symbol, "According to Sociologist, the male and female secret has an external as well as internal aspect. To elevate himself to a higher plan of thought and existence, man should grasp the meaning of the concept 'Ardhanarisvara'.[60]

Now let us proceed with the other misinterpreted symbol that is Yajña.

(c) Yajña : Sacrifice :

The first two discussed symbols linga and Ardhanarisvara are attached with sex notion. The third symbol which we are going to discuss is also partially related with it. The name of the symbol, as it is mentioned above is Yajña or sacrifice.

Tantra is way of sublimation from gross to subtle. According to Tantra, the pleasure which comes out from the physical copulation can be sublimated into the spiritual bliss. This is the real import of the Symbol Yajña.

Before going into the root, let as first see the etymological meaning of the term Yajña.* yaj is the root verb of this term which stands for propitiation.[61] For Tantra every act is a propitiation or worship of the Higher Reality. Even the action like copulation which we generally consider as low is viewed with veneration. Now let us see how this Yajña is performed externally and internally.

In the external formation of sacrifice, an altar is formed out from special materials and by experts. Burning fire is placed inside the altar. During the performance of Yajña, clarified butter is constantly poured into the sacrificial fire. Sometimes animals are also used as an object of oblation for the satisfaction of diety. The Yajña takes place in the physical body. According to Tantra, body is an altar in which the some or elixir is being constantly dropped from the Sahasràr Cakra or brain. This elixir is being consumed by the fire situated in the navel region or the Manipura Cakra. Semen is the gross form of elixir or sona which is ejected maximum in quantity in intercourse. Constant or frequent section of semen naturally results into decay because semen is the very base of life. A Tàntric Sàdhaka retains this consumption through the Kundalini yoga or other Tàntric practises. This is the real Tàntric yajña which takes place within the body with the result that Sàdhaka enjoys the immortality.

Tàntric notion of yajña also leads one from the individuality to the universality. The concept of Yajña is the core of the Sàdhànà aspect. In Sàdhanà, Sadhaka offers many objects like flowers, lamp of fire, fragrant powder, various types of corns namely Till, Cooked rice, Java, milk etc. But in Tantra Sadhana there is no need to offer all these things in gross form. Because a Sadhaka mentally offers all the five elemental forces or the five gross elements (Panca Mahàbhùta) namely Earth (Prithvi), Water (Àp), Fire (Teja), Vàyu (Air) and Ether (Àkàsa) in the place of flower, lamp, powder etc. Whatever he does physically that is not important in Tantra Sàdhanà but he is mentally attuned with the universe and offers it to desired diety. This kind of yajña removes the boundary of limitations and Sàdhaka feels identity with the entire cosmos.

Now let us see what seems objectionable to lay man in this symbol. As we have mentioned, in Sacrifice, sometimes animals are also offered. But Tantra has never taken the gross animals. This misinterpretation happens due to lack of proper knowledge of Tàntric meaning of animal. The Tantra like Yogini Tantra, Anadakalpa etc. have clearly mentioned that the animals like vice should be killed with the sword of knowledge.[62] From this reference we can say without having doubt that if we take the real meaning of ablation, there is nothing objectionable. On the contrary the proper view leads one to the infinite from finite or from individuality to universality.

Now apart from these symbols, which are largely related with sex concept, there are also some symbols which are highly significant in the Tàntric Sàdhanà. Among them, Symbol of 5 M's is the basic one. Now let us see about it.

(d) Panca makara: 5 M's:

The misinterpretation of the Symbol 5 M's plays prominent role in the degeneration of the Tàntric tradition and system. In Tantrism, there are also some sub-sects namely, Vàmàcàra, Daksinàcàra, Divyacara etc. Among them 5 M's. comes under the title Vamacara. Let us see first why it is known as 5 M's. It is known as so because either are five items in it start with the syllable 'M' that is why it is recognized as 5 M's. These are namely Madya (Wine), Màmsa (meat), Matsya (Fish), Mudrà (Grain) and Maithuna (Copulation). Let us see each of the syllable respectively.

i. *Madya—Wine:*

Madya means wine. The inherent quality of Madya is to make man aloof from the outer world. To forget the frustration created from the machine age, man resorts to take wine, which gives him temporary relief.

Madya is not utilized in Tantra in the sense of wine. In Tantra madya is not a liquor but as the Kulàrnava Tantra declares, it is an energy.[63] All of us have a treasure of energy which is hidden in our body. Tantra shows the approach of awakening of it. Sàdhaka, who awakens the centres of energy (Cakra) releases his senses from the engrossment (Pàsa) of the outer world. The utilization of this Tàntric

Madya results into not in a temporary relief as it so happens in the gross wine but it gives life-time bliss to the Sàdhaka. By doing so he yokes his self with his original nature, that is Siva or limitless infinite element. The peculiarity of Tàntric madya is that, as the Kulàrnava Tantra declares it leads Sàdhaka to Brahman.[64] or a state known as Bràhmi sthiti (*i.e.* identity with ultimate Reality).

Hence for Tantra, Madya is not a wine and Tantric Sàdhaka is not a drunkard but he is a worshipper of Sakti or energy.

ii. *Màmsa—Meat:*

The meaning of Màmsa is meat. It is meat. It is one of the seven components of the body i.e. rakta (Blood), Rasa (Essence), Màmsa (Meat), Majja (Veins), Asthi (Bone), Sukra (Semen) and Meda (Marrow). Meat is utilized for food purpose by animals as well as human beings. But how this meat is related with Tantra ?

In the Tantric pujà, meat of an animal, sometimes of a human being also is offered to a deity for the satisfaction of diety. But to utilize a gross meat is not consistent with the Tàntric meaning of meat. What is then the Tàntric meaning of meat one may question.

Generally, we get meat by killing the animal. In Tantra whenever the term animal is used, lit does not indicate animal like goat, donkey, deer etc. In Tantra, man in a natural state is considered as Pasu or an animal. To sacrifice this animal means to raise man from his natural state to a Supra natural state or even to the spiritual state. Offering meat means process of sublimation, from gross to subtle. According to the kulàrnava Tantra those who does so is the real eater of meat and rest are the killers of life.

So Tantra has never favoured the killing of any gross animal but one has to kill his animal like gross instincts.

iii. *Matsya-Fish:*

Matsya stands for fish. In Tantra it symbolically represents mind and prana, the Vital force.

As fish floats in the water, mind also floats in the sea of sense objects. Mind always moves from one sense object to the other and due to its constant movement it loose its powers. So far the channelization of mental powers, according to the Tantra, mid should be a entrapped by the net of Sàdhanà.*

The another subtle meaning of Matsya is prana or vital force. Vayu (air) is the gross form of it. As has been explained in the Heaths yoga pradipika, mind and pràna follow one another. By controlling the one, another can automatically be controlled.* So here like mind, pràna is also considered as fish. But how Tantra considers prana as fish one may wish to know.

According to the Tantra, though prana pervades in the entire body; we breath, which is the grossform of pràna through right and left nostrils which in terms of Tantra known as Pingala, the sun and Idà, the moon respectively. In the Yougic terms, life span depends upon the amount of Pràna consumed through respiration. The more amount of it we utilize, we can enjoy more life or longevity. Pràna floats either in Pinglà or in Idà which we feel it in the form of respiration. So to minimize the amount of respiration or in other words to enjoy longevity one has to control the prana, which moves like a fish in Idà and pingla.

From this we can conclusively say that the Tàntric meaning of Matsya is totally different from the gross one.

iv. *Mudrà—Grain:*

Mudrà means grain or cooked food. The root verb of Mudrà is mud means to please.[67] We eat food for the sustenance of life without which our body can not persist. Food nourishes body and with the result body becomes healthy and with healthy body, we enjoy all pleasures.

Tantra has not taken only the gross meaning of Mudrà. According to it, in the realm of Sàdhanà, the spiritual body of a Sàdhaka should be strengthened by the spiritual food like Jñàna Vairagya, Tapa etc. The Tantra tattava prakàsa has mentioned eight types of Mudra or grain like desire, greed, anger, greed anger, lust etc..., which should be cooked or sublimated into the fire of Brahman.[68]

This is the real food of Sàdhaka by which he sustains his spiritual life. So this is the Tàntric meaning of Mudrà.

Mudrà also is a part of Tantra Sàdhanà and there it is a means for identifying spiritually various parts of the body with cosmic force or energy. So in Tantra, Mudra is not merely a cooked food but it also contains spiritual meaning.

v. *Maithuna- Copulation:*

Maithuna indicates copulation. Copulation is an union of male and female; the opposite poles required to be brought together for the purpose of creation by nature.

Tantra has presented the subtle meaning of creation, that is, spiritual creation for which two opposite poles are required. These two poles are Siva and Sakti. Siva resides at the Sahasrara (brain) while Sakti at the Mùlàdhàra Cakra (pelvic region). In between these two there are six centres of energy around the spinal cord. The energy which resides at the Mùlàdhàra Cakra awakens and penetrates all the centres and unites with Siva at the Sahasràra Cakra. This is the real Tàntric maithuna or copulation which occurs in the Sàdhka.[69]

So it is not a gross maithuna or copulation taking place between two physical bodies but it is a spiritual communion with Siva and Sakti which gives birth or transforms the whole personality of a Sadhaka.

With the help of Tàntric treatise, we have tried to see the correct meaning of Tàntra symbols. Tantric way of Sadhana is so effective which gives quick results. So to avoid misuse of it, this system is armoured in the symbolic terminology. So symbols are designed to maintain its secrecy. But due to lack of its proper knowledge, a distortion takes place into the Tantra system.

We could see from the description, of the symbol that there is a World-wide difference between a gross meaning and a Tàntric meaning. The symbols like linga, Ardhanàrisvara, Maithuna etc. are largely distorted because of their relevance with sex notion. We consider sex as a cause degeneration but as the Kulàrnava says that which brings about degeneration can as well be a means for sublimation.[70] Thus the subtle meaning of symbol is enough to decide its soundness.

F. Conclusion:

Body is the only means for achieving any goal. Disease proves to be obstacle in the path of gaining the goal. Tantra is a Sàdhanà, system. In the way of Sàdhanà, Sàdhaka has to face many physical disorders and mental disturbances. Tantra has not over looked this fact. To come out from this, it has mentioned certain processes which are designed for strengthening body mind complex and thereby fortifying the instrument for achieving all goals physical as well as supra physical.

If we glace over the content of the first chapter with a view to examine the therapeutic aspect of it, will be found highly significant. The very definition of Tantra reflects its therapeutic aspect. As we have seen, one of the meaning of Tantra according to the Sabdakalpadruma is medicine (ousadhi). The other meaning liberation is also deal with this aspect. It liberates Sàdhaka from the physical and mental ailments. How Tantra does this that we have already indicated as and when we have found an opportunity. Still however by way of stating the investigations we have found clearly, we would like to recapitulated briefly as follows:

Tantra does this by two ways: One by the cultivation of strong will power and second, by the utilization of pàrad or mercury and its preparations.

As has been accepted, generally everybody has got its own medicine, that is, its power of inbuilt resistance against attacks from disease. This can be further cultivated by the cultivation of strong willpower. From the principles of Tantra we could see that, Tantra Sàdhanà is nothing but the awakening of inner powers of senses, body and mind. Willpower is the key of all powers. With the cultivation of it, one can open doors to the other latent powers. The power of resistance against diseases is also included within it.

Tantra also does this same job by the utilization of mercury (pàradà) and its preparations. Mercury is considered as highly medicinal metal. But is can not be used in a natural form because of its poisonous nature. Tàntric seers have found out this fact five thousand years back and also worked out the process (Samskàra) to make mercury fit for medicinal use.

Lord Siva is considered as the originator of this process of alchemy who is also the reveller of Tantra. With the help of these two only a Hatha yogi or a Tàntric Sàdhaka survived on the snowy summits of mountains without having any antibiotic drugs. This is but the physical side of Tàntric way of dealing with bodily ailments. We now turn to its mental side.

G. Symbol and their therapeutic value:

As is the case with Pàrada or mercury in strengthening body so also, Tantra has a distinct medicine for mental ailments. And it is surprising to note that Tantra uses psychological symbols or linguistical alphabets as symbols for curing the mental diseases by cultivating inner potent mental powers.

Symbols are also highly significant in this regards in lying stress on mental aspect. Mind plays prominent role in mental and physical diseases. Mental disturbances are expressed sometimes in a physical disorders or physical disturbance sometimes makes mind weak. Thus all our diseases are psycho-somatic. Being a subtler than body, mind's effect on body is felt more powerful. Tantra has recognized this fact much earlier than we started talking about psycho-somatic aspect of disease.

The Tàntrics prescribe the use of symbol for making mind calm and positive by concentrating it on syllables or figures of particular types. It is undisturbed and concentrated mind which is a source of creative imagination or all the creativity of mind. Tàntric Sàdhanà is based on imagination. Sàdhaka has to positively think that he is offering this or that object. This positive thinking also helps as therapy if the mind is diseased. The theory of auto-suggestion in psychology is highly related with this aspect. In the process of auto-suggestion patient gives strong suggestion or he imagines himself quite healthy very powerfully. This process gives relief to patient and gradually helps in curing himself from diseases. Tàntric Sàdhanà through symbols strengthens the positive powers of imaginations which Sàdhaka can utilize as a therapy for himself and also can be used as therapeutic means for curing others.

FOOT NOTE

1. Tan, Tanyate, Pànini, vi, 4, 44—to extend, to spread. Taken from the dictionary of Sir Monier Williams, p. 435, Oriental Publishers, Delhi-6.

2. Tanyate Vistàryate Jànan anena iti Tantram. Cited by Shri Ram Sharma, Tantra Vijñàna (Hindi), Part I, p. 171. Published by Samskrit Sansthana.

3. In the Tantra Sàdhanà, there is a Mantra in which Sàdhaka or a practitioner mentally offers the earth element of the universe as a fragrance of flower. (Lam Prithvitàtt vatmakam gandham parkalpayàmi) Like wise he offers all the five elements of the universe in his worship. In doing so, he has to expand his area of imagination as far as possible till he mentally offers the entire universe to his desired deity.

4. Singh, Lalan Prasad. Tantra: Its Mystic and Scientific basis, p. 1, Concept Publishing Company. Delhi 1976.

5. Tanute Tràyate Nityam Tantramitham Vidurbudhahà.I H.P. Sastri. Nep II, p. 69. Cited by Shree Chakravarti, Chintaharan, Tantras—studies on their religion and literature, p. 2, Punthi Pustak, Calcutta-4, 1963.

6. Tanoti Vipulànarthàn tattvamantram samnvitàm Tranam cakurute yasmàt tantramithamabhidhtyate. Kamika Tantra, Cited by Shah Dhirajlal T. Tàntro nu. Tàrana (Gujaràti), Jain Sàhitya Mandir, 1961.

7. Tanoti tanyate iti và I Ousadhi, Sidhànta Sabdakalpadruma, Part II, pp. 584-85, Motilal Banarsidas, Delhi, 1961.

8. Geden A. S., Encyclopedia of Religion and Ethics, Edited by Hastings, Vol. 8, p. 193, Vol. XII.

9. Sàrìrakamimanàsà bhàsya of Samkaràcàrya. Commentry on the Brahma Sutra 2.2.32 Sarvathànu papattesca I

10. Àgamonama àñityupsargàta gam dhatoh aca pratyaye nisapannah tantra Sastrarupoartha avabodhakah I

11. Àgatam Pancavakatràtta gatam ca girijànane I
Matam Ca vàsudeasya tasmàt Àgamaucyate

12. Singh, Lalan Prasad. Tantra—Its Mystic and Scientific basis, p. 2. Concept Publishing Company, Delhi, 1976.

13. Avalon, Arthur, Principles of Tantra, Part I, p. 99, Preface. Ganesh and Co., Madras, 1969.

14. Dasgupta, Shashi Bhusan, Aspects of Indian Religious Thought, p. 148. A. Mukherjee and Co., Calcutta 1957.

15. Kundu, Nundo Lall, Non-Dualism in Saiva and Sàkta philosophy, p. 3 (Who has cited from Preface to pre-historic ancient Hindu-Indian by Donald A. Mackenzie) Sri Bhairabi Jogeswari Math, Calcutta.

16. Ghose, N. N., Early history of India, p. 17. The Indian Press (Pub.) Private Ltd., 1960, Fourth edition.

17. Singh, Lalan Prasad, Tantra—Its Mystic and Scientific basis, p4. Concept Publishing Co., Delhi 1976, First Edition.

18. Review of Ram Chandra Rao's book 'The truth about Tantra' by S. K. Ram Chandra. Published in 'The Times of India', April 19, Sunday, 1981.

19. Kundu, Nundo Lall, Non-Dualism in Saiva and Sàkta philosophy, p. 8. Sri Bhairabi Jogeswari Math, Calcutta.

20. Ghose N. N., Early history of India, p. 16. Indian Press (Pub.) Private Ltd., Allahabad, 1960, Fourth Edition.

21. Krite Srutyuktàchàrastretàyàng Smrtisam-bhavah I

Dvàpare tu purànoktang Kalau àgamlakevalam II

Taken from the Principles of Tantra, Arthur Avalon, Part I, p. 36, Introduction. Ganesh and Company.

22. Arthur Avalon, Principles of Tantra, Part I, p. 48. Ganesh and Company.

23. Chakravarty, Chintaharan, 'The Tantras Studies on their religion and literature', p. 2. Punthi Pustak, Calcutta 1963, First Edition.

24. Singh, Lalan Prasad, Tantra—Its Mystic and Scientific basis, p. 9. Concept Publishing Company, Delhi 1976, First Edition.

25. Ibid., p. 9.

26. Avalon, Arthur, Principles of Tantra, p. 110, Part I. Ganesh and Company, Madras, 1969, Fourth Edition.

27. Chambers Twentieth Century dictionary. Edited by A. M. Macdonald B.A. (O'xan), p. 1035, Allied Publishers Private Ltd., 1974.

28. Sivasaktyoh jàyàpatinyàyena jàyayà Saktya Yuktascat prapancarupasantanam nirmàtum Saknoti, tayà viyuktascet na Sknoti iti

29. Tvam màtà sarva bhùtànàm pità caaham Sanàtanah I

Dvyosca yo raso devi mahà maithuna sambhavah II

Rasàrnava Tantra. Edited by Panta, Tarànanda, Patal I, p. 34. Chaukhamba Sanskrit Series, 1939.

30. Mookerji, Ajit, Tantra Asana—A way to self-realization, p. 62. Published by Ravi Kumar, 1965, First Edition.

31. Mama rùpàsi devi tvam na bhedosti tvyà mama I

The Mahànirvàna Tantra. Edited by Avalon, Arthur, Chaps. 1-95, p. 9. Motilal Banarasidas, Delhi, Reprinted 1977.

32. Sivasyàbhyàntare Saktih Sakterabhyantarah Sivah I

Antarm naiva jàniyàccandracandrikayoriv.

Siddha-Siddhànta-Paddhati and other works of the Nàth Yogis. By Smt. Mallik, kalyani. Upadesa-4-26, p. 21. Poona oriental Book House, Poona, 1954.

33. Sivahsaktyà yukto yadi bhavati Saktah Prabhvitum na cedevam devo na kualu kusalah Spanditymapi I

Sundrya Lahari Verse—I. Sri Sañkara Bhagavatpàdàchàrya. Edited by Kuppuswami, A. The Ministry of Education & Social Welfare, Government of India, 1976.

34. Yasmin tyaktà Mahàkali Saktihìnàh Sadàsivah I

Saktyà yuto yadà devi, tadaiv Sivarùpakah I

Saktihine Savah Sàksàt purusatvam na muncati II

Todal Tantra, taken from karpùra Stavaràja (Hind) by Mahàkàla, p. 60.

Motilal Banarsidas.

35. Swami Prabavananda. The Sipritual Heritage of India, pp. 14-45.

Georage Allen and Unwin Ltd., London, 1962, First Edition.

36. Mookerji, Ajit. Tantra Asana—A way to self realization, p. 16. Published by Ravikumara, 1965. First Edition.

37. Deha devàlayo devi jivo devah Sadàsivah I

The Kulàrnava Tantra. Ullasa—9-41.

38. Visvasàra Tantra. Cited by Avalon, Arthur. Principles of Tantra, Part I, p. 118, Ganesh and Company, 1969.

39. Ajñàna granthibhedo yah-Sa moksa iti Kathyate I

Sarvajñabhairava Tantra. Taken from Lupta àgama Samgraha.

40. Bhàvastu mànaso dharm Sabdasya hi Katham bhavet. Nigama Kalpananda. Cited by Dikshit, Sadasiva in Karpùra Stava Ràja of Mahakala, p. 84, Motilal Banarsidas.

41. Mana eva manusyànàm Kàranam bandha moksayoh I

Yathaivalingità Kàntà tathaivaliñgità Sutà I

Dharma Sàstra. Quoted in the Karpùra Stava Ràja, p. 34.

42. Ata eva yada yasya bhavana kutsita bhavet I

Tada dosaya bhavati nanyatha dusanam Kvacit.

Kaulavali Tantra. Cited in karpura Stava Raja, p. 34.

43. Yaireva patanam dravyaih Siddhihitaiheva Caudità I

The Kulàrnava Tantra. 5-48.

44. Bhogo yogàyate Sàksàt patakam sukrutàyate

Moksàyate ca Sansàrah Kuladharma Ku klesvari I

Ibid. 2-24.

45. Danielou, Alain. Hindu Polytheism. Routledge and Kegan Paul. London. 1964. First Edition.

46. Vastumàtram tu yaddrasyam Samsàre triguna hi tat II 69 II Drasyam ca nirgunam loke na bhùtam no bhavisyati I Nirgunah Parmàtmàssou na tu drsyah Kadàcana II 70 II

Vyàs, Krusna Dwaipàyana. Srimad Devi Bhàgavatam. 3.6.69-70. Edited by Pandey Ràmateja Pandita Pustakàlaya, Kàshi 1956.

47. Gavàm Sarvàñajam Ksìram Streveta Stana-Mukhàd Yatha I

Tathà Sarvagato devah pratimàdisu ràjate II

The Kulàrnava Tantra 6-75.

48. Liyate gamyate yatra yena sarvam caracaram II
Tadetadliñgamitiyuktam liñgatattva paràyanaih I
Layagatyartha yohetuhùtatvat Sarvadehinam II
Lingamitiucyate Sàksàtsivah Sakalaniskalah II Anubhava Sùtram.
Adhikaran—3. Verse 3-4. Yogatantra-Granthmala (3) Edited by Shukla, Badrinath Part-I. Varanaseya Sanskrit Visva Vidhyalya, first Edition 1970.

49. a) Liñgat Sarvam Samutpannam Layam tasmin PrakìrtitamI
Vàtul Suddhàkhyà Tantra 1-51.
b). Linge tu jàyate Sarvam jagat Sthavàrajangam II
Ibid. 1-72.
Taken from Yogatantra-Granthmàlà (3), p. 181.

50. Liñga Sabdena Vidvànsah Srustisamhàra Kàranam I
layàdàgamanàccahubhàvànam padama vyam I
Tantrakaloka-4/131.
Mrucchailadhatyratnàdibhvam linga na pùjayet I
Yajedadhyàtmikam liñgam yatra linam Caràcram
Bahiliàgasya liñgatvamanenàdhisthitam yatah
Tantraloka—5/120
Mishra, Janardana, Bhàrtiya Pratika Vidyà, pp. 106, 107, Bihara Rastrabhasa Parisada, Patnà, 1959.

51. Lokam Liñgvamakam Jñàtva liñga Yostpyate hi màma I
Na me tasmàt priyatarah Priya ka Vidhyate Kvacita
Shiva Puràna.

52. Layam gacchati bhùtàni Samsàre nikhil yatah I
srustikàle punah Srutihtasmàt liñgamudà hatam II
Linga Puràna.

53. Danielou, Alain. Hindu Polytheism, p. 127, Routledge and Kegan Paul.

54. Ibid.

55. Sivasaktyoh jàyàpatinyàyena Jàyayà Sàktya Yuktasceta prapancarùpa Santànam nirmàtum Saknoti.

Saundrya Lahari, Vàcyàrtha of the First Verse, p. 2.

56. Lingam Siva iti jñeyath pìthath Saktihi udàhàta I

Yoni liñgaprakàrena jagatsrustayartha Karanam II

The Vàtul Suddhàkhya Tantra, 1-69.

57. Zimmer, Henrich. "Myths and Symbols in Indian art and civilization, p. 127. Edited by Joseph Campbell. The Bollingen Series, VI. 1946.

58. Etàdi manusyatvàvicchinnàdi bhedàhà Vàmàbhàge mama aksunna nivàsah I

Evam tad Buddhe Svayameva nirdesàh iti ardhanàri Svaratvena mahapuruso Vidyate I

Tripur Samhità. Translationand Verse taken from the Great Yogic Sermon by Majithia Surendra Singh, p. 32, Allied Publishers, 1969.

59. Mookerji, Ajit, Tantra Asana—A way to self realization, p. 57. Published by Ravi Kumar, First Edition, 1965.

60. Majithis Surendra Singh, 'The Great Yogic Sermon', p. 32.

61. yaj = μ worship or propitiate. Samskruta Sabdàrtha Koustabha.

Edited by Sharma, Dwàrkàprasàd, p. 948, Ramnàràyana Làl Beniprasàda, Third Edition.

62. Punyàpunya pasum hatvà jñàna khadagena yogivata I yogini Tantra.

Sri Ram Sharma. Tantra mahàvijñàna (Hindi), Part I, p. 253.

63. Surà Saktih Sivo mamsam tadbhoktà bhairavah svyam I

The Kulàrnava Tantra 5.79.

64. Madirà brahmagàh proktah cittsodhana Sàdhanà I

The Kulàrnava Tantra 5-41.

65. Manasà caindriyaganam Samyamyàtmani yojayet I

Taken from Tantra Mahàvijñàna (Hindi), Sharma, Sri Ràma,p. 261.

66. Cale vàte calam cittam niscale niscalam bhavet I

The Hatha yoga Pradipikà 2.2. Translated into English by sinh, Pancham, p. 13. Oriental Books Reprint Corporation, 1975.

67. Mudam Kurvanti devànàm manànsi dràvayanti ca I

Tasmànmudrà iti khyàtà darsitavyàh Kulesvari.

The Kulàrnava Tantra 17-57.

68. Àsatrusnàjugupsàbhaya Visdaghrunàmànalajjà prakopàh I

Brahmàgnavasta mudràh parasukrutijanah pacyamànàh samantàt I

Tantra Mahàvijñàna, Sri Ràma Sharma, p. 264, Part I (Hindi), Samskruti Samsthàna, Bareli.

69. Paràsktiyàtma maithunam samyogànanda nirbhara

The kulàrnava Tantra 5-112.

70. Yaireva Patanam dravyaih Siddhilitaih eva caudità I

Ibid 5-48.

CHAPTER 2

Supernatural Power, Buddhist and Hindu

By Yogi C.M. Chen

1. Supernatural Power, Buddhist and Hindu

We Buddhists give most of our attention to the practice of concentration and meditation on voidness, through this, all the sorrows and the root of sorrow, which is the inner self, the eighth consciousness, may be overcome and transformed into Buddha's wisdom. We are not desirous of getting supernatural powers that will make the inner self strong enough to fight with others. When the farmer works diligently in the field and it is time for harvest, the chaff is gotten along with the rice; so we practice according to tantric instructions for full Enlightenment in this lifetime and when we become accomplished, supernatural powers are also attained simultaneously. But to the Western scholars or researchers, supernatural power is an interesting subject. They read books on Tantric Hinduism which describe many wonderful things and think that the Hindus certainly have no less power than the Tantric Buddhists. In order to correct this misunderstanding, I am writing this chapter.

The main difference in this regard is this—the Tantric Hindus and other non-Buddhists have five supernatural powers: divyacaksus (instantaneous view of anything anywhere), divyasrotra (ability to hear any sound anywhere), paracittajnana (ability to know the thoughts of all other minds), purvanivasanusmrtijnana (knowledge of all former existences of oneself and others), and rddhisaksatkriya (the power to be anywhere or do anything at will). But only the Buddhist has the final one, Anasrava, which accompanies all the others. With Anasrava, the above mentioned powers become limitless and greater in power. The reason for the Buddhist superiority is this: the Buddhist Tantric practitioner spends much time and energy avoiding his own sorrows whether gross or subtle. The root of sorrow is ignorance and the root of ignorance is the inner self. The Tantric Hindu, holding tightly to the higher self, limits his wisdom and power while the Buddhist, being free of even this, attains unlimited wisdom and power.

Enough of theory. Let us look at some actual comparisons. We can begin with the scriptures. A. In Hinduism, in the book Mysterious Kundalini by Vasant G. Rele, on page 68, eight Ashta siddhis are written of:

> (1) "Anima—A yogi concentrating, meditating and fixing his attention on this quality of the soul during forced exhalation, draws together his entire energy to a point which is then made to penetrate into all bodies so as to make them vibrate according to the will of the Yogi."

But he cannot again draw his energy from this little point into the voidness nature which is the final truth of Buddhism. He does not believe in that.

> (2) "Mahima—This is also a special quality of the soul. A yogi by mere inhalation of air makes his body assume a large size and comprehends the universe in himself as was done by Krishna."

This universe spoken of is the worldly one and does not include that of Buddhism, and he cannot enlarge and extend himself from his universe to the voidness nature because of the same reason given in the last Siddhi. It is said in the philosophy of mathematics that infinity and the unlimited decimals are equal to zero, so the voidness can be both infinity and unlimited decimals. The Hindus have no anasrava supernatural power and they cannot reach voidness.

> (3) "Laghima—He can make his body as light as a feather so that it can float in the air or in water. The yogi's power of traveling thousands of miles in a moment is attributed to this Siddhi."

Even traveling in a moment is limited by time. In Buddhism there are many good examples of this power, one of which was quoted in "Kundalini Yoga" (a Hindu work by Sivananda) as follows: "Once an outsider asked Milarepa for a contest to see which of them could arrive at the top of the snow hill first.

This outsider is riding on a magic drum and begins to fly up the hill the next morning while Milarepa was still sleeping. When his disciple saw the outsider halfway up the hill, he called for Milarepa to get up but Milarepa continued to sleep. The outsider had almost arrived at the top of the hill. By only one thought Milarepa arrived at the top. The outsider lost all his supernatural power and fell down." Here Milarepa, though quoted by a Hindu worker, is well-known even to Westerners as the Great Tibetan Yogi. To a great yogi accomplished in the voidness meditation, there is no limitation in space and time, but to a Hindu there is the limitation of Brahma or the high self which I have mentioned in practically every chapter.

> (4) "Garima—A yogi increases specific gravity of the body thus making it as heavy as a mountain by swallowing large draughts of air and compressing them in the tissues of the body."

The quantities of air swallowed cannot compare with that of the Tantric Buddhist.

> (5) "Prapti—When in Samadhi the yogi acquires the power of predicting future events, of understanding unknown languages, of curing disease and of divining the unexpressed thoughts of others."

The time of the future is limited by the kapla of Brahma's creation and destruction, but a Buddhist is free from it.

> (6) "Prakamya—It is the containing of more than one's expectations and the power of casting off the old skin and maintaining a youthful appearance for an unusually long period of time. This is recorded as being true in the case of yogi King Yayati and Aleiluades who maintained unfading youth to the last day of their lives."

Here we read that he has a last day, but there are great Buddhist yogis such as the lotus-born Padmasambhava who are still alive. Not only he but many, many others such as Saraha, Harvarapa, Biwapa, and females Such as Nukuma, Yishitoga,

Sukarsiddhi who have attained non-death Enlightenment.

(7) "Vasitva—It is the power of taming living creatures and bringing them under control."

This occurs in Tantric Buddhism also. Even in Ch'an there are disciples who were tigers. In Christianity Saint Francis tamed a fox who had killed many people.

(8) Ishitva—Obtaining universal dominion either in this life or in the next by means of yoga."

The dominion of their universe belongs to this world, and is only equal to the iron cakravartin of Buddhism. There are still higher ones such as copper, silver and gold. The last one conquers those before it.

B. In "Kundalini Yoga" there are also mentioned twenty-six minor siddhis which I have quoted below:

1. Freedom from hunger and thirst. 2. Freedom from the effects of heat and cold. 3. Freedom from raga-dwesha. 4. Doora Darshan, clairvoyance or doora-drishti. 5. Doorasravan clair-audience or doora-sruti and doora-pravachana. 6. Manojaya—control of the mind. 7. Kama-rupa—the yogi can take any form he likes. 8. Parakaya pravesha—he can enter into another body, can animate a dead body and enter into it by transferring his soul. 9. Iccha mrityu—death at his will. 10. Devanam Saha krida and darshana—playing with devas after seeing them. 11. Yatha sankalpa—he can get whatever he likes. 12. Trikala jnana—knowledge of the past, present and future. 13. Advandva—beyond the pairs of opposites. 14. Vak siddhi—whatever the yogi predicts will come to pass by practice of satya, prophecy. 15. The yogi can turn base metal into gold. 16. Kaya Vyuha—taking as many bodies as the yogi likes to exhaust all his karma in one life. 17. Darduri siddhi—having the jumping power of a frog. 18. Pat ala siddhi—the Yogi becomes lord of desires, destroys sorrows and diseases. 19. He gets knowledge of his past life. 20. He gets knowledge of the cluster of stars and planets. 21. He gets the power of perceiving the siddhis. 22. He gets mastery of

the elements and mastery of prana. 23. Kamachari—he can move to any place he likes. 24. He gets omnipotence and omniscience. 25. Vayu siddhi—rise in the air and stay above the ground. 26. He can point out the place where hidden treasures lie.

The above twenty-six siddhis are very common to Buddhism in the exoteric and esoteric schools. All those siddhis, even though the twenty-sixth one bears the same name as it does in Tantric Buddhism, are limited by Brahma.

C. If we compare the supernatural power of the Tantras in both religions we will find that the power of the exoteric school is produced from meditation of Samadhi but that of the esoteric school is produced from both Samadhi and untying the lotuses (chakras). There is no mention of supernatural powers being produced from untying lotuses in "Kundalini Yoga", but in "The Serpent Power" by Sir John Woodroffe we find a few verses on this subject. Below I quote from a few Hindu works on this matter. 1. Shatchakra Nirupana, verse 13, states, "By meditating thus on Her who shines within Muladhara chakra, with the lustre of ten million suns, a man becomes Lord of speech and King among men and an Adept in all kinds of learning. He becomes ever free from all diseases, and his inmost spirit becomes full of great gladness. Pure of disposition by his deep and musical words, he serves the foremost of the Devas." But in Tantric Buddhism, the supernatural power derived is as stated above in addition to which the yogi gets the accomplishment of the excellent view of voidness corresponding to the stage of beholding the truth and gets all Supernatural powers of the first and second stages of a Bodhisattva called the greatly rejoicing (Pramudita). These powers as described in the Avatamsaka Sutra are: a) Achievement in one hundred kinds of samadhis, which are more profound than the eight stages of heavenly dhyanas. b) The ability to see one hundred Buddha worlds. c) The ability to shake one hundred Buddha worlds. d) The ability to know the secret power of one hundred Buddhas. e) The ability to pass over one hundred Buddha worlds.

f) The ability to convert one hundred world's people. g) The ability to live in one hundred Kalpas h) The ability to know the beginning and the end of one hundred kalpas. i) The ability to enter into one hundred victorious Dharmagates. j) The ability to appear in one hundred incarnations, and k) each incarnation is able to appear with one hundred families around him.

A Tantric Buddhist will never lose those powers. The second stage of power is one thousand fold more than this first stage.

2. Concerning the Svadhisthana chakra, verse 18 of the same book states: "He who meditates upon this stainless lotus, which is named Svadhisthana is freed immediately from all his enemies, such as the fault of egoism and so forth. He becomes a Lord among Yogis and is like the Sun illuminating the dense darkness of ignorance. The wealth of his nectar-like words flows in prose and verse in well-reasoned discourse." When the svadhisthana chakra of a Tantric Buddhist is open he obtains the supernatural powers of the third and fourth stages besides those mentioned above. The third and fourth stages of supernatural powers areone hundred thousand fold more than those of the first stage.

3. Verse 26 discusses the power of Manipura chakra as follows: "He who meditates on this Heart Lotus becomes the Lord of Speech and (like) Ishvara he is able to protect and destroy the worlds." We quote from verse 27, "Foremost among Yogis, he ever is dearer than the dearest to women. He is preeminently wise and full of noble deeds. His senses are completely under control. His mind with its intense concentration is engrossed in thoughts of Brahman. His inspired speech flows like a stream of water. He is like the Devata who is beloved of Lakshrni and he is able at will to enter another's body." Including the above powers, the Buddhist gets all the powers of the fifth and sixth stages which are more than one million times that of the first stage.

4. The Anahata chakra is discussed in verse 31, "He who

has attained complete knowledge of the Atma, becomes by constantly concentrating his mind on this lotus, a great Sage, eloquent and wise and enjoys uninterrupted peace of mind. He sees the three periods and becomes the benefactor of all, free from diseases and sorrow and long-lived and, like Hamsa, the destroyer of endless dangers." The Tantric Buddhist gets the supernatural powers of the seventh and eighth stage of a Bodhisattva which are countless times more than the first stage and attains the wisdom of Sambhogakaya. He also gets four kinds of unlimited interpretations (Pratisamvid).

5. The discussion of the powers of the Ajna chakra is in verse 34 of this same Shatchakra Nirupana: "Meditation of this lotus enables one to quickly enter another's body at will and become the most excellent among Munis (sages) and all knowing and seeing. He becomes the benefactor of all and versed in all Shastras. He realizes his unity with Brahman and acquires excellent and unknown powers. Full of fame and long-lived, he ever becomes the Creator, Destroyer and Preserver, of the three worlds." In addition to these the Buddhist obtains the powers of the ninth and tenth stages of the Bodhisattva. There are no other powersthat can be compared with them except Buddha.

6. Concerning the supernatural powers of the Sahasrara chakra, verse 45 states: "That most excellent of men who has controlled his mind and knows this place is never again born in the world, wandering as there is nothing in the three worlds which binds him. His mind being controlled and his aim achieved, he possesses complete power to do all he wishes and moves toward the Brahman. His speech, whether in prose or in verse, is ever pure and sweet." The Tantric Buddhist also gets full Enlightenment of Buddhahood in this lifetime. Not only the highest position in the exoteric school but also that in the esoteric school which is the great-pleasure-wisdom-body (Mahasukha-PrajnaKaya) in Vajrayana.

D. There are ten excellent secret powers of a Buddha which give complete knowledge of the following:

1. What is right or wrong in every condition.

2. What is the karma of every being, past, present and future

3. All stages of Dhyana liberation and Samadhi.

4. The powers and faculties of all beings.

5. The desires or moral direction of every being.

6. The actual condition of every individual.

7. The direction and consequence of all Dharmas.

8. All causes of mortality and of good and evil in their reality.

9. The end of all beings and Nirvana.

10. The destruction of all illusions of every kind.

E. There are ten wonders or incomprehensibilities of Buddha. They are in two groups: the traceable or manifested, and the original. The traceable ones are:

1. The incomprehensible surrounding—the universe, sphere or whole embracing mind, Buddha and all things as a unity.
2. The incomprehensible wisdom—a Buddha's all-embracing knowledge arising from such a universe.
3. The incomprehensible deeds—his deeds expressive of his wisdom.
4. The incomprehensible stages—his attainment of all the various Buddha's stages such as the ten stages of a Bodhisattva.
5. The incomprehensible Dharmas—the three Dharmas of truth, wisdom and vision.
6. The incomprehensible response—his response to appeals because "All beings are my children."

7. The incomprehensible supernatural power—we have already mentioned these.

8. The incomprehensible preaching.

9. The incomprehensible supernatural retinue.

10. The incomprehensible blessings—for a universal elevation to Buddhahood.

The original group of incomprehensibilities are:

1. The incomprehensible initial impulse or causative drive of Buddhahood.

2. The incomprehensible result or fruit in eternity, joy and purity.

3. The incomprehensible realm.

4. The incomprehensible response.

5. The incomprehensible supernatural powers.

6. The incomprehensible preaching.

7. The incomprehensible retinue.

8. The incomprehensible Nirvana.

9. The incomprehensible life.

10. The incomprehensible blessings.

G. There are eighteen special characteristics of a Buddha which are different from Bodhisattvas. They are:

His perfection of 1. the body, 2. mouth or speech, 3. memory, 4. impartiality to all, 5. serenity, 6. self-sacrifice, 7. unceasing wisdom in it, desire to save all, 8. unflaggin zeal therein, 9. unfailing thought thereto, 10. wisdom in it, 11. power of deliverance, 12. the principles of it, 13. revealing perfection and wisdom in deed, 14. in words, 15. In thought, 16. perfect knowledge of the past, 17. present, 18. future.

H. In brief the Tantric Buddhist can have the same powers

as the Tantric Hindu and infinitely more. You may ask why it is that at the same chakra the powers of the yogi may be different. It is because the wisdom-energy and the median nerve and the wisdom drops are different from one another. Those powers of the Tantric Hindu are like heavenly ones, but those of the Buddhist is of Buddhahood which is beyond heaven without the limitation of Brahma. Please review Chapters 3 and 6 of "Discrimination between Buddhist and Hindu Tantras." Furthermore, in our method of the holy flame rising up and the wisdom drops descending, the Buddhist yogi gets the four holy pleasures, which accompany the truth of voidness such as: The first pleasure accompanies the equilibrium voidness, the second pleasure accompanies wide or vast voidness, the third accompanies the great voidness and the fourth accompanies the all voidness. These four kinds of voidness are the source of unlimited supernatural power which is not in agreement with the high self of Hinduism.

I. All of the statements concerning supernatural powers are true in a very real and concrete sense, but to the Western scholar who has no experience in practice, they seem like abstractions. Therefore, let me introduce an historical story which shows the comparison of the power of Buddha and the gurus of the six schools of non-Buddhism.

Once Sudatta put all of his gold on the land of the garden of the benefactor of orphans (who owned the land) in order to exchange his gold for a temple for Buddha Gautama. The envious and selfish gurus of the six non-Buddhist schools then asked Sudatta for a contest in which the powers of the disciples of the Buddha would be compared with those of their schools. If the Buddhists won, they could build the temple, but if they lost they could not build the temple. Sudatta was very grieved. Sariputra, the disciple of Buddha Gautama heard this and consoled him saying, "Suppose they had enough gurus to fill the world, they could not move a hair of mine." Sudatta asked his father, King of Sravasti, to strike the golden drum to call together all the great people of Sravasti who were eighteen million in number. Among these, three million belonged to the six non-Buddhist schools.

Sariputra sat in Samadhi and thought, "If in my past lives I was very grateful to my parents and very faithful to the Buddhist monks and Brahmans, then today they should pay me respect when they meet me at the assembly." As a result of his good karma, all of the gurus and their disciples who were three million in number, bowed down to him without their willfully wanting to do so just as the grass bows down to the wind. This welcome actually occurred.

Among the disciples of the six schools, there was a well known one named Loututza who was very skilled in supernatural powers. First, he performed some magic on the ground and immediately a tree grew up with different flowers and fruits on it. The audience said, "It is made by Loututza." Then Sariputra made an elephant appear which had six tusks. On each of these there were seven lotuses, and on each lotus there were seven female angels sitting. The elephant went to a pool and drank all the water leaving the pool dry. The audience then said, "The victor is the sage Sariputra. How can Loututza be compared with him?" Then with shame, Loututza made a magic mountain which was adorned with seven kinds of gems. On the mountain were many trees with flowers and fruits. From his samadhi, Sariputra sent out a vajra. He held it in his hand and pointed it toward the distant magic mountain. It became dust at once. The audience was surprised and asked again, "How can Loututza be compared with the sage?" Loututza made a flying dragon and caused gems to rain from the sky and brought on a clap of loud thunder. Sariputra sent a kind of Garuda to eat the dragon. The audience said, "To compare powers with a Buddhist sage is only to harm oneself." Loututza made an unusually large magic bull with a large body, big feet and big horns. Sariputra sent a lion who instantaneously ate the bull leaving no remains. Angrily, Loututza transformed himself into a powerful Yaksha body with flaming hair, red eyes, four long incisors and emiting fire from his body toward the sage. Suddenly, Sariputra transformed his body into that of Vaisravana, King of Yakshas. Loututza feared his king and backed away to escape punishment, but the fire permeated all four directions. There was no escape. All he could do was to bow down before Sariputra and take refuge from him. After

Loututza embraced Sariputra as his guru and many disciples from the six schools of non-Buddhists were converted, the Buddhist sage manifested many supernatural powers. I do not have the time to write them here because now I want to introduce the supernatural powers of Buddha Gautama.

J. Even though King Bimbisara was converted to Buddhism, his brother still believed in the six non-Buddhist gurus. In vain the king had many times advised his brother to become a Buddhist. It was the habit of this brother to give alms to all monks regardless of religion. The following story relates what happened on one occasion when the supernatural powers of Gautama Buddha and those of the six non-Buddhist gurus were compared.

The six gurus and their disciples had gathered to receive alms. The Buddha with his disciples purposely arrived late and the only seats left were those that were in the low section. Because of the Buddha's noble virtue and Supernatural power, all six gurus and disciples unwillfully moved to the lower part, and although they tried to return to the high section, the seats remained those of the low section. The patron began to give water for washing from the higher section to the lower but Buddha humbly said, "Please give it to your guru first." Those six gurus became dumb. They could only raise their arms to point to Gautama who sat in the seat of the higher section, far in the distance from them. The Buddha's prayer was as music. When the food was finally served, Buddha repeated that the patron's guru should be served first, but the food flew to the top of the gurus heads where they could not reach it. Upon Buddha's receiving the food, each of the others also received their food.

After the meal, the patron asked Buddha to preach but he declined suggesting that the six gurus be asked first. They became dumb and could not preach. Then Buddha preached and the patron, his officials and family were all converted. With a grieved countenance and an envious mind each guru went back to his own church and learned some methods of magic. A demon transformed himself into a human body and taught them how to obtain more powers than they had before. Then these gurus asked the king whether they might have another opportunity to compare their powers with those of the Buddha. After receiving the Buddha's permission, the king made all preparations, but Buddha wanted all the people of five Indian lands to witness his victory, so when all the peoples of one province had gathered, he moved on to Vaisali, then to Kausambi or Vatsapattna in central India, and finally to a place called Sravasti which was controlled by the well-known king Prasenajit. Gautama manifested many kinds of supernatural powers in the Dharma assembly where India's peoples gathered. The six gurus, however, were unable to do anything. It is a rule that outsiders can do no magic in the presence of a Buddha.

For many, many days the Buddha preached to his audience. While Indra stood on the left side and Brahma himself stood on the right. Both were the protectors of Buddha. Indra offered Buddha a lion seat. At the moment he sat there was a sacred sound which emitted from the five vajras and struck down all six gurus. They threw themselves into the water. Although in different tongues the peoples of India gave praise to Buddha Gautama as the victor and final Lord. This story can be found in the "Good and Evil Sutra". It is a trustworthy record.

K. Now you will say that the above story was with regard to Buddha and the six gurus but I have said nothing about Buddha and Brahma, the highest of all higher selves. I will quote from the Madhyamagama Sutra.

Once Buddha knew by his parocitta-jnana (ability to know

the thoughts of all other minds) that the perverse view (Mithya) had arisen in Brahma's mind that all is permanent. Buddha flew to Brahma's heaven and after explaining that everything is impermanent, converted Brahma. Brahma then requested competition of their powers which Buddha agreed to. First Brahma magically hid his body but wherever he went Buddha could see him and said, "You are here, you are there." Brahma could not elude such magic. Then Buddha said, "I will try to hide myself, please try to point out where I am." Buddha then hid his body in voidness meditation. On purpose he let Brahma hear his voice, but Brahma could not point him out. Thereby Brahma's faith was increased.

I don't know what Tantric Hindus of today think of this story. Would they have more power than Brahma? Your Lord Brahma has already been converted, so what are you waiting for now?

My good readers, I must beg your pardon. It is not that I really wanted to write such a long chapter on supernatural powers, but only that I know you are so interested. Buddha's powers were so many that even those magic verses of his "Retractable Penis Sutra" are greater than those found in the Rig-Veda. Since I cannot introduce this sutra here in its entirety, I cannot help but stop here.

As the village beauty is charming not only in her ornaments but in her nature, so is the Buddha's excellent virtues not only in his Supernatural powers but in his samadhi of voidness, in his Bodhi-heart and his wisdom.

CHAPTER - 3

TANTRA AND NIRVAN

CHAPTER - 3

1. Who Seeks Nirvàna ?

THE LATER Buddhist change of attitude toward the final goal is paralleled exactly by the contemporary Hindu development. As we have seen,[1] in Hìnayàna usage the term *bodhisattva* denoted a great being on the point of becoming a Buddha and so passing from time to nirvàna, an archetype of the Buddhist lay-initiate escaping from the world, whereas in the Màhàyana the concept was translated into a time-reaffirming symbol of universal saviorship. Through renouncing Buddhahood the Bodhisattva made it clear that the task of moksa, "release, liberation, redemption from the vicissitudes of time," was not the highest good; in fact, that moksa is finally meaningless, samsàra and nirvàna being equally of the nature of sùnyatà, "emptiness, the void." In the same spirit the Hindu Tàntric initiate exclaims: "Who seeks nirvàna ?" "What is gained by moksa ?" "Water mingles with water."

This point of view is rendered in many of the conversations of Srì Ràmakrishna with his lay disciples.

"Once upon a time," he told them one evening, " a sannyàsin entered the temple of Jagganàth. As he looked at the holy image he debated within himself whether God had a form or was formless. He passed his staff from left to right to feel whether it touched the image. The staff touched nothing. He understood that there was no image before him; he concluded that God was formless. Next he passed the staff from right to left. It touched the image. The sannyàsin understood thsat God had form. Thus he realized that God has form and, again, is formless."[2]

"What is vijñàna ?" he said on another occasion. "It is knowing God in a special way. The awareness and conviction that fire exists in wood is jñàna, knowledge. But to cook rice on that fire, eat the rice, and get nourishment from it is vijnana. To know by one's inner experience that God exists is jñàna. But to talk to Him, to enjoy Him as Child, as Friend, as Master, as Beloved, is vijñàna. The realization that God alone has become the universe and all living beings is vijnana."[3]

And with respect to the ideal of becoming annihilate in Brahman, he would sometimes say, quoting the poet Ràm-prasàd, " I love to eat sugar, I do not want to become sugar."[3a]

The Mahàyàna Bodhisattva tastes unending saviorship by devoting himself with absolute selflessness to his teaching task in the vortex of the world; in the same spirit, the Hindu Tàntric initiate, by persevering in the dualisitc attitude of devotion *(bhakti)*, enjoys without cease the beatitude of the knowledge of the omnipresence of the Goddess.

"The Divine Mother revealed to me in the Kàlì temple that it was She who had become everything," Srì Ràmakrishna told his friends. "She showed me that everything was full of Consciousness. The Image was Consciousness, the altar was Consciousness, the water-vessels were Consciousness, the doorsill was Consciousness, the marble floor was Consciousness- all was Consciousness. I found everything inside the room soaked, as it were, in Bliss-the Bliss of Satcidànanda.[4] I saw a wicked man in front of the Kàlì temple; but in him also I saw the Power of the Divine Mother vibrating. That was why I fed a cat with the food that was to be offered to the Divine Mother."[5]

"The jñàni, sticking to the path of knowledge," he explained again, "always reasons about the Reality, saying, "Not this, not this.' Brahman is neither 'this' nor 'that'; It is neither the universe nor its living beings. Reasoning in this way, the mind becomes steady. Then it disappears and the aspirant goes into samadhi. This is the Knowledge of Brahman. It is the unwavering conviction of the jñàñi that Brahman alone is real and the world illusory, llike a dream. What Brahman is cannot be described. One cannot even say that Brahman is a Person. This is the opinion of the jñànìs, the followers of Vedànta philosophy.

"But the bhaktas accept all the states of consciousness. They take the waking state to be real also. They don't think the world to be illusory, like a dream. They say that the universe is a manifestation of God's power and glory. God has created all these-sky, stars, moon, sun, mountains, ocean, men, animals. They constitute His glory. He is within us, in our hearts. Again, He is outside. The most advanced devotees say that He Himself has become all this-the twenty-four cosmic principles, the universe, and all living beings. The dev-otee of God wants to eat sugar, not to become sugar. *(All laugh.)*

"Do you know how the lover of God feels ?" Ràmakrishna continued. "His attitude is 'O God, Thou art the Master, and I am Thy servant. Thou art the Mother, and I am Thy child.' Or again: 'Thou art my Father and Mother. Thou art the Whole, and I am a part.' He doesn't like to say, 'I am Brahman.'

"The yogì seeks to realize the Paramàtman, the Supreme Soul. His idea is the union of the embodied soul and the Supreme Soul. He withdraws his mind from sense-objects and rites to concentrate it on the Paramàtman. Therefore, during the first stage of his spiritual discipline, he retires into solitude and with undivided attention practices meditation in a fixed posture.

"But the Reality is one and the same. The difference is only in name. He who is Brahman is verily Àtman, and again, He is the Bhagavan, the Blessed Lord. He is Brahman to the followers of the path of knowledge, Paramatman to the yogis, and Bhagavan to the lovers of God.

"The jñànis, who adhere to the nondualistic philosophy of Vedanta, say that the acts of creation, preservation, and destruction, the universe itself and all its living beings, are the manifestations of Sakti, the Divine power.[6] If you reason it out, you will realize that all these are as illusory as a dream. Brahman alone is the Reality, and all else is unreal. Even this very Sakti is unsubstantial, like a dream.

"But though you reason all your life, unless you are established in samàdhi, you cannot go beyond the jurisdiction of Sakti. Even when you say, 'I am meditating,' or 'I am contemplating,' still you are moving in the realm of Sakti, within Its power.

"Thus Brahman and Sakti are identical. If you accept the one, you must accept the other. It is like fire and its power to burn. If you see the fire, you must recognize its power to burn also. You cannot think of fire without its power to burn, nor can you think of the power to burn without fire. You cannot conceive of the sun's rays without the sun, nor can you conceive of the sun without its rays.

"What is milk like ? Oh, you say, it is something white. You cannot think of the milk without the whiteness, and again, you cannot think of the whiteness without the milk.

"Thus one cannot think of Brahman without Sakti, or of Sakti without Brahman. One cannot think of the Absolute without the Relative, or of the Relative without the Absolute.

"The Primordial Power is ever at play.[7] She is creating, preserving, and destroying in play, as it were. This Power is called Kàlì. Kàlì is verily Brahman, and Brahman is verily Kàlì. It is one and the same Reality. When we think of it as inactive, that is to say, not engaged in the acts of creation, preservation, and destruction, then we call It Brahman. But when It engages in these activities, then we call it Kàlì or Sakti. The Reality is one and the same; the difference is in name and form."[8]

This introductory exposition of the Tàntric point of view was given on the deck of a little excursion-steamer, sailing up and down the Ganges, one beautiful autumn afternoon in 1882. Keshab Chandra Sen (1838-84), the distinguished leader of the semi-Hindu, semi-Christian Brahmo Samàj,[9] had come, with a number of his following, to visit Srì Ràmakrishna at Dakshineswar, a suburb of the modern city of Calcutta, where the saintly teacher was serving as priest in a temple dedicated to the Black Goddess, Kàlì. Keshab was a modern, occidentalized Hindu gentleman, with a cosmopolitan outlook, and a sàttvic, humanistic, progressive religious philosophy-not unlike that of his New England contemporary, the Transcendentalist (and student of the *Bhagavad Gità*), Ralph Waldo Emerson. Ràmakrishna, on the other hand, was a thorough Hindu-intentionally ignorant of

English, nurtured in the traditions of his motherland, long-practiced in the techniques of introverted contemplation, and filled with the experience of God. The coming together of these two religious leaders was a meeting of the modern, timely India and the timeless-the modern consciousnes of India with the half-forgotten divine symbols of its own unconscious. Noteworthy, moreover, is the fact that on this occasion the teacher was not the Western-educated, tailored gentleman, who had been entertained in London by the Queen, but the yogì in his loincloth, speaking of the traditional Indian Gods out of his own direct experience.

KESHAB *(with a smile)*: "Describe to us, sir, in how many ways Kàlì, the Divine Mother, sports in this world."

SRI RÀMAKRISHNA *(also with a smile)*: "Oh, She plays in different ways. It is She alone who is known as Mahà-Kalì ["The Great Black One"], Nitya-Kàlì ["The Everlasting Black One"], Smasàna-Kàli ["Kàlì of the Cremation Ground"], Raksà-Kàlì ["Goblin Kàlì"], and Syàmà-Kàlì ["Dark Kali"]. Mahà-Kàlì and Nitya-Kàlì are mentioned in the Tantra Philosophy. When there were neither the creation, nor the sun, the moon, the planets, and the earth, and when darkness was enveloped in darkness, then the Mother, the Formless One, Mahà-kàlì, the Great Power, was one with Mahà-Kàlì [this is the masculine form of the same name], the Absolute.

"Syàmà-Kàlì has a somewhat tender aspect and is worshiped in the Hindu households. She is the Dispenser of boons and the Dispeller of fear. People worship Raksà-Kàlì, the Protects, in times of epidemic, famine, earthquake, drought, and flood. Smasàna-Kàlì is the embodiment of the power of destruction. She resides in the cremation ground, surrounded by corpses, jackals, and terrible female spirits. From Her mouth flows a stream of blood, from Her neck hangs a garland of human heads, and around Her waist is a girdle made of human hands.

"After the destruction of the universe, at the end of a great cycle, the Divine Mother garners the seeds for the next creation. She is like the elderly mistress of the house, who has a hotch-potch-pot in which she keeps different articles for the house-hold use. *(All laugh)*, Oh, yes ! Housewives have pots like that, where they keep sea-foam, blue pills, small bundles of seeds of cucumber, pumpkin, and gourd, and so on. They take them out when they want them. In the same way, after the destruction of the universe, my Divine Mother, the Embodiment of Brahman, gathers together the seeds for the next creation. After the creation the Primal Power dwells in the universe itself. She brigs fotrth this phenomenal world and then pervades it. In the Vedas creation is likened to the spider and its web. The spider brings the web out of itself and then remains in it. God is the container of the universe and also what is contained in it.

"Is Kàlì, my Divine Mother, of a black complexion ? She appears black because She is viewed from a distance; but when intimately known She is no longer so. The sky appears blue at a distance; but look at air close by and you will find that it has no color. The water of the ocean looks blue at a distance, but when you go near and take it in your hand, you find that it is colorless."

Srì Ràmakrishana, filled with lover for the Goddess, then sang to her two songs of the Bengali devotee and yogì Ràmprasàd, after which he resumed his talk.

"The Divine Mother is always sportive and playful. This universe is Her play. She is self-willed and must always have her own way. She is full of bliss. She gives freedom to one out of a hundred thousand."

A BRÀHMO DEVOTEE: "But, sir, if She likes She can give freedom to all. Why, then, has She kept us bound to the world ?"

SRÌ RÀMAKRISHNA: "That is Her will. She wants to continue playing with Her created beings. In a game of hide-and-seek the running about soon stops if in the beginning all the players touch the `granny'. If all touch her, then how can the game go on? That displeases her. Her pleasure is in continuing the game.

"It is as if the Divine Mother said to the human mind in confidence, with a sign from Her eye, `Go and enjoy the world." How can one blame the mind ? The mind can disentangle itself from worldliness if, through her grace, She makes it turn toward Herself."

Singing again the songs of Ràmprasàd, Sri Ràmakrishna interrupted his discourse, but then continued. "Bondage is of the mind, and freedom is also of the mind. A man is free if he constantly thinks: 'I am a free soul. How can I be bound, whether I live in the world or in the forest ? I am a child of God, the King of Kings. Who can bind me ?' If bitten by a snake, a man may get rid of its venom by saying emphatically, 'There is no poison in me.' In the same way, by repeating with grit and determination, 'I am not bound, I am free,' one really becomes so-one really becomes free.

"One someone gave me a book of the Christians. I asked him to read it to me. It talked about nothing but sin. *(To Keshab Chandra Sen:)* Sin is the only thing one hears of at your Brahmo Samàj, too. The wretch who constantly says, 'I am bound, I am bound,' only succeeds in being bound. He who says day and night, 'I am a sinner, I am a sinner,' really becomes a sinner.

"One should have such burning faith in god that one can say: 'What ? I have repeated the name of God, and can sin still cling to me ? How can I be a sinner any more ? How can I be in bondage any more ?

"If a man repeats the name of God, his body, mind, and everything become pure. Why should one talk about sin and hell, and such things ? Say but once, 'O Lord, I have undoubtedly done wicked things, but I won't repeat them.' And have faith in his name."

Sri Ràmakrishna sang:

If only I can pass away repeating Durgà's name;
How canst Thou then, O Blessed One,
Withhold from me deliverance,
Wretched though I may be ? . . . . . .

Then he said: "To my Divine Mother I prayed only for pure love, I offered flowers at Her Lotus Feet and prayed to Her: 'Mother, here is Thy virtue, here is Thy vice. Take them both and grant me only pure love for Thee. Here is Thy knowledge, here is Thy ignorance. Take them both and grant me only pure love for Thee. Here is Thy purity, here is Thy impurity. Take them both, Mother, and grant me only pure love for Thee. Here is Thy dharma, here is Thy adharma. Take them both, Mother, and grant me only pure love for Thee."[10]

In Tantra the theistic attitude practically obliterates the abstract ideal of the Formless Brahman *(nirguna brahman)* in favor of Brahman-in-the-Gunas *(saguna brahman)* - the Lord *(Ìsvara)*, the personal God; and the latter is represented by the Tantrics preferably in the female aspect, since in this the nature of Màyà-Sakti is most immediately affirmed.[11] The Tàntric development supported the return to power in popular Hinduism of the figure of the Mother Goddess of the innumerable names- Devì, Durgà, Kàlì, Pàrvatì, Umà, Satì, Padmà, Candì, Tripura-sundàri, etc.-whose cult, rooted in the Neolithic past, had been overshadowed for a period of about a thousand years by the male divinities of the patriarchal Àryan pantheon. The Goddess began to reassert herself in the period of the later Upanisads.[12] She is today the chief divinity again. All the consorts of the various gods are her manifestations, and, as the sakti or "power" of their husbands, represent the energy that has brought the latter into manifestation. Moreover, as Mahàmàya, the Goddess personifies the World Illusion, within the bounds and thralldom of which exist all forms whatsoever, whether gross or subtle, earthly or angelic, even those of the highest gods. She is the primary embodiment of the transcendent principle, and as such the mother of all names and forms."God Himself," states Ramakrishna, "is Mahàmàyà, who deludes the world with Her illusion and conjures up the magic of creation, preservation, and destruction. She has spread this veil of ignorance before our eyes. We can go into the inner chamber only when She lets us pass through the door."[13] It is entirely possible that in this reinstatement of the Goddess, both in the popular cults and in the deep philosophy of the Tantra, we have another sign of the resurgence of the religiousity of the non-Àryan, pre-Àryan, matriarchal tradition of Dravidian times.

The Tàntric movement differs from Jainism and Buddhism, however, inasmuch as it adheres to the authority of the Vedas, seeking rather to assimilate and adjust itself to the orthodox tradition than to exclude and refute it. In this it parallels the patttern of popular Hinduism. Indeed, the mixture of Tàntric and Vedàntic traits in modern HIndu life, ritual, and thought is so intìmate that they present themselves as an organic whole. The Tantrics speak of their texts as "The Fifth Veda," "The Veda for This Iron Age." "For the first of the four world ages, *sruti* (Veda) was given; for the second, *smrti* (the teachings of the sages, Dharamasastra, etc.), for the third, *puràna* (the epics, etc.), and for the fourth, *àgama* (the Tantric texts)."[14]

As has been pointed out by Sir John Woodroffe, whose studies are the most important examinations of the Tantra published in modern times: "The Sàkta followers of the Àgama claim that its Tantras [i.e., "books"] contain the very core of the Veda...As men have no longer the capacity, longevity and moral strength required to carry out the Vaidika Karma-kanda [the ritual section of the Veda], the Tantra Sàstra prescribes a Sàdhanà [religious discipline] of its own for the attainment of the common end of all Sastra, that is, a happy life on earth, Heaven thereafter, and at length Liberation."[15]

Both the Tantra and popular Hinduism accept the truth of Advaita Vedànta but shift the accent to the positive aspect of màyà. The world is the unending manifestation of the dynamic aspect of the divine, and as such should not be devaluated and discarded as suffering and imperfection, but celebrated, penetrated by enlightening insight, and experienced with understanding. The hair of the Goddess is dishevelled in her frantic, self-maddened dance which produces the mirage of samsàra, but the perfect devotee is not thereby dismayed. "Though the mother beat him," says Ràmprasàd, "the child cries `Mother' ! O Mother,' and clings still tighter to her garment."[16] The Vedàntic yogì never tires of stating that *kaivalya*, "isolation-integration," can be attained only by turning away from the distracting allure of the world and worshiping with single-pointed attention the formless Brahman-Atman; to the Tàntric, however-as to the normal child of the world-this notion seems pathological, the wrong-headed effect of a certain malady of intellect . By the true lover of the Goddess, not merely the seeking of liberation but even its attainment is not desired. For what is the use of salvation if it means absorption ? "I like eating sugar," as Ràmprasàd said, "but I have no desire to become sugar."[17] Let those who suffer from the toils of samsàra seek release: the perfect devotee does not suffer; for he can both visualize and experience life and the universe as the revelation of that Supreme Divine Force *(sakti)* with which he is in love, the all-comprehensive Divine Being in its cosmic aspect of playful, aimless display *(lìlà)_which* precipitates pain as well as joy, but in its bliss transcends them both. He is filled with the holy madness of that "ecstatic love" *(prema)* which transmutes the world.

> This very world is a mansion of mirth;
> Here I can eat, here drink and make merry.[18]

Artha (prosperity), kàma (the fulfillment of sensual desires), dharma (the enactment of the religious and moral rituals of everyday life, with an acceptance of the burden of all the duties), and moksa (release from it all) are one. The polarity of moksa and the trivarga[19] is transcended and dissolved not in introverted realization alone, but in living feeling as well. Byi virtue of his talent of lover for the merciful Goddess, the true devotee discovers that the fourfold fruit of artha , kama, dharma, and moksa falls into the palm of his hand.

"Come, let us go for a walk, O mind, to Kàlì, the Wish-ful-filling Tree," wrote Ràmprasàd; "And there beneath It gather the four fruits of life."[20] "The mind ever seeks the Dark Beautiful One, he states again. "Do as you wish. Who wants Nirvana ?"

Tàntrism, as a matter of course, insists on the holiness and purity of all things; hence, the "five forbidden things" ("the five M's, as they are called) constitute the substance of the sacramental fare in certain Tantric rites: wine *(madya)*, meat *(màmsa)*, fish *(matsya)*, parched grain *(mudrà)*,[21] and sexual intercourse *(maithuna)*. As in the parallel Mahàyàna initiations,[22] the nondualist realization makes all the world one-one, holy, and pure. All beings and things are members of a single mystic "family" *(kula)*. There is therefore no thought of caste within the Tàntric holy "circles" *(cakra)*. Sùdras, outcastes, and Brahmans alike are eliegible for initiation-if spiritually competent. The aspirant must only be intelligent, with his senses controlled, one who abstains from injuring any being, ever doing good to all, pure, a believer in the Veda, and a nondualist, whose faith and refuge are in Brahman: "Such a one is competent for this scripture; otherwise he is no adept."[23]

One's secular social standing is of no consequence whatsoever within the sphere of the truly spiritual hierarchy. Moreover, women as well as men are eligible not only to receive the highest initiation but also to confer it in the role of guru. "Initiation by woman is efficacious; that by the mother is eightlfold so," we read in the *Yoginì Tantra*.[24] In striking contrast to the Vedic texts, wherein even the hearing of the Veda is forbidden to a sùdra, and wherein women are consigned to a secondary (though highly praised and sentimentalized) sphere of spiritual competency and aspiration, the Tantras transcend the limits of social and biological differentiation.

However, it must not be supposed that this indifference to the rules of caste implies any idea of revolution within the social sphere, as distinguished from the sphere of spiritual progress. The initiate returns to his post in society; for there to, is the manifestation of Sakti. The world is affirmed, just as it is-neither renounced, as by an ascetic, nor corrected, as by a social reformer. The prerequisite to the initiation being an actual superiority to fear and desire, and the rite itself a confirmation of the understanding that all is divine, the true lover of the Goddess remains content with what She has bestowed, not finding fault with the various traditional proprieties of time and place, but beholding the Divine power, with whom he is himself identical in essence, within all arrangements.

For the idea of dharma is intrinsic to Indian thought. The sacrament of the "five forbidden things" does not open a way to either libertinism or revolution. On the plane of ego-consciousnes, where one operates as an individual member of society, the dharma of one's caste and àsrama[25] still prevails, the height beyond dharma and adharma being ascended only by one in whom the mind has been transcended-in which superior state there can be no question of a desire to enjoy the benefits of illegal practices. The Tàntric ritual of wine, meat, fish, parched grain, and sexual intercourse is accomplished not as a lawbreaking revel, but under the cautious supervision of a guru, in a controlled state of "nondualist" (advaitic) realization, and as the culminating festival of a long sequence of spiritual disciplines, through many lives. The spiritual emotion of the adept is *prema*: ecstatic, egoless, beatific bliss in the realization of transcendent identity.

Coming down again from this sublime height of form-annihilating realization to the kingdom of phenomenality, differentiation is seen but there is no estrangement; there is no tendency then to deprecate-for there is no guilt, there has been no Fall. The world does not require to be reformed; nor are its laws to be disregarded. All of the various planes of manifestation of the absolute can be beheld in a dispassionate spirit. The solid, the liquid, and the gaseous states of the one substance, under differing conditions, producing differing effects, are accepted without moral or emotional preference. For the whole spectacle of the world, without exception, is generated by the dynamism of Màyà-Sakti, the power of the cosmic dance *(lìlà)* of the dark and terrible, sublime, all-nourishing and consuming Mother of the World. The beings of the world, and all the ranges of experience, are but waves and strata in a single, ever-flowing, universal stream of life.

Obviously, this is the view that we have already encountered many times in our present examination of the philosophies of India. The hymn from the *Taittirìya Bràhmana*, celebrating the substance and energy of the world as food,[26] was based on a nondualism of just this kind. The released-reborn celebrates himself as food-and-eater; for though the gross outer sheath of the organism, the "sheath of food" *(annamayakosa)*, is not the whole of the divine manifestation (there being, in the subtle sphere of the several inner sheaths, more subtle formations and incarnations of the Supreme Essence), nevertheless "food is not to be despised." The reality of Brahman was realized in the orthodox Vedic Brahman tradition progressively, under various manifestations: as the life-matter of the material world, in the Hymn of food; or as the sun, "he who yonder glows," in a multitude of other Brahmanic songs of celebration; or again, as the macrocosmic life-breath *(vàyu)*, "he who blows," which is the counterpart of the microcosmic *prana*.

Throughout the history of Bràhman thought there has been a reiterated assertion-either violent and passionate, or vigorously controlled-that the "One is both at once," and in this respect Tàntrism continues the orthodox Vedic line. Everything proceeds from the same supernal source. All beings are members of a single holy family, proceeding from the one and only divine substance. And this view involves, as we have seen, on the one hand devaluation of the peculiarly personal nuances of individuality, but on the other a bold affirmation of all that may ever come to be. Màyà, the world illusion, is not to be rejected but embraced. The lyricism of the Vedànta-Gìtàs[27] gave expression to this world-affirmative. The Tantra does so again. And it is reflected today through the whole range of the popular Hindu theologies.

But there is a peculiar and essential trait of the Tàntric Yea which distinguishes it from the earlier philosophies-or at least these as they appear in the orthodox texts and commentaries; for the ideal of Tàntrism is to achieve illumination precisely by means of those very objects which the earlier sages sought to banish from their consciousness. The ancient Vedic cult was world-affirmative, but its rites were primarily those of the vast popular and royal ceremonials in honor of the gods of the macrocosm; they did not invite one to fathom the deep resources of the microcosm. The forest philosophers, on the other hand-devoted to the introvert techniques of Jainism, Yoga, Sànkhya, Vedànta, and the Hìnayàna-strove to repress their personal biological impulses by subjecting themselves to a spiritual reducing diet for the conquering of rajas, tamas and the vasanas (the vessels of memory and desire); and when this transferred them finally to a plane beyond sin and virtue-they remained virtuous. Indeed, they had had to cast away the capacity for sinning at the very start, as the first prerequisite of their approach to a guru.[28] But in the Tantra, whereas the goal is that of the meditating yogì (not worldly power, such as was sought by the ancient Bràhman conjurers of the forces of the universe, but enlightenment, absolute consciousness, and the beatitude of transcendental being), the manner of approach is that , not of Nay, but of Yea. That is to say, the world-attitude is affirmative, as in the Veda, but the gods are now addressed as dwelling within the microcosm.

Thus it may by said that if the Vedànta seems to represent the conquest of the monistic Àryan Brahman heritage by the dualist ideology of the pre-Aryan seekers of integration-isolation *(kaivalya)*,[29] in the Tantra we are, perhaps, justified in recognizing just the opposite influence; a rerendering of the pre-Àryan problem of psychophysical transubstantiation in terms of the nondual philosophy of the all-affirmative Bràhmanic point of view. Here the candidate for wisdom does not seek a detour by which to circumvent the sphere of the passions-crushing them within himself and shutting his eyes to their manifestations without, until, made clean as an angle, he may safely open his eyes again to regard the cyclone of samsara with the untroubled gaze of a disembodied apparition. Quite the contrary; the Tantric hero *(vira)* goes directly *through* the sphere of greatest danger.

It is an essential principle of the Tantric idea that man, in general, must rise through and by means of nature, not by the rejection of nature, "As one falls onto the ground," the *Kularnava Tantra* states, " so one must lift oneself by the aid of the ground,"[30] The pleasure of love, the pleasure of human feeling, is the bliss of the Goddess in her world-productive dance, the bliss of siva and his sakti in their eternal realization of identity; only as known in the inferior mode of ego-consciousness. The creature of passion has only to wash away his sense of ego, and then the same act that formerly was an obstruction becomes the tide that bears him to the realization of the absolute as bliss *(ànanda)*. Moreover, this tide of passion itself may become the baptizing water by which the taint of ego-consciousness is washed away. Following the Tàntric method, the hero *(vìra)* floats beyond himself on the roused but canalized current. This is what has discredited the method in the eyes of the community. Its heroic acceptance, without quibble, of the full impact and implication of the nondual celebration of the world as Brahman has seemed far too bold, and too sensational, to those whose view of saintliness embrances of Lord's transcendent repose but omits the detail of His mystery play *(lìlà)* of continuous creation.

A right method cannot exclude the body;. for the body is *devatà*, the visible form of Brahman as jìva. "The Sàdhaka [the Tàntric student !," writes Sir John Woodroffe, "is taught not to think that we are one with the Divine in Liberation only, but here and now, in every act we do. For in truth all such is Sakti. It is siva who as Sakti is acting in and through the Sàdhaka...When this is realized in every natural function, then, each exercise thereof ceases to be a mere animal act and becomes a religious rite—a Yajña. Every function is a part of the Divine Action (*sakti*) in Nature. Thus, when taking drink in the form of wine the Vira knows it to be Tàrà Dravamayì, that is, 'the Saviour Herself in liquid form.' How (it is said) can he who truly sees in it the Saviour Mother receive from it harm ?... When the Vìra eats, drinks or has sexual intercourse, he does so not with the thought of himself as a separate individual satisfying his own peculiar limited wants, an animal filching as it were from nature the enjoyment he has, but thinking of himself in such enjoyment as Siva, saying 'Sivo 'ham,' 'Bhairavo' ham' ('I am siva)."[31]

Sex, in Tàntrism, has a high symbolic role. The holy fear of the uncontrollable forces in human nature and the consequent strict resistance to the animal instincts and energies, which characterize the common history of man from the earliest taboo to the latest moral tract, can be explained as the result and residue of devastating experiences in the past of the race and the by-product of the successful, historical struggle for independence of a higher, "purer', spiritual principle. The primitive forces, out of the depths of which this principle arose, like the victorious sun, Sol Invictus, climbing the heavens out of the stormy sea (the turbulent abode of the monsters of the deep), had to be checked, held at bay and tied back, like the Greek Titans imprisoned under volcanic Aetna, or like the great Dragon of the Revelation of St. John. The very real peril of an elementary upheaval and rocking outburst led to the construction of protective dichotomic systems, such as those, not only of jainism and the Sàñkhya, but also of the Persian Zoroastrian ethical religion, the Gnosis of the Near East, Christianity, Manichaeism, and the usual codes of manners of primitive and civilized mankind. In India, in the ancient world, and among most of the peoples known to anthropologists and historians, there has been, however, an institutionalized system of festivals —festivals of the gods and genii of vegetation—whereby, without danger to the community, the conventional fiction of good and evil could be suspended for a moment and an experience permitted of the mighty titan-powers of the deep. Carnival, the day of masks, revealing all the odd forms that dwell in the profundities of the soul, spills forth its symbols, and for one dreamlike, nightmarish, sacred day, the ordered, timid consciousness freely revels in a sacramentally canalized experience of its own destruction.

The masks are dreamlike. Dreamlike also are the carnival events. Indeed, the world of sleep into which we descend every night, when the tensions of consciousness are relaxed, is precisely that from which the demons, elves, divine and devilish figures of the world mythologies have all been derived. All the gods dwell within us, willing to support us, and capable of supporting us, but they require the submission of consciousness, an abdication of sovereignty on the part of our conscious wills. In so far, however, as the little ego regards its own plans as the best, it resists rigorously the forces of its divine substratum. The gods thereupon become dangerous for it, and the individual becomes his own hell. The ancient people made made peace with the excluded forces by holding them in worship and allowing them their daemonic carnival—even while cultivating, simultaneously, under the forms of sacrifices to the higher gods, a fruitful relationship with the forces implicated in the social system. And by this means they won the permission, so to speak, of their own unconscious to continue in the conventional conscious attitude of profitable virtue.

But the Tàntric sàdhaka is not interested in conventional survival so much as in the fathoming of life and the discovering of its timeless secret. Hence the makeshift of carnival is not enough; for this only supports the general illusion. His goal is to incorporate the excluded forces as well as those accepted generally, and experience by this means the essential nonexistence of the antagonistic polarity-its vanishing away, its nirvana; i.e., the intrinsic purity and innocence of the seemingly dark and dangerous sphere. In this way he breaks within himself the tension of the "forbidden," and resolves everything in light; recognizing in everything the one Sakti which is the general support of the world, macrocosmic as well as microcosmic, the mother of the gods and elves, the weaver of the moon-dream of history. Therewith comes release from the world-illusion-release through its full enjoyment or realization.

Hence the great Tàntric formula (so different from that of the earlier Hindu yogic disciplines): yoga (the yoking of empirical consciousness to transcendental consciousness) and bhoga ("enjoyment," the experience of life's joy and suffering) are the same, Bhoga itself can be made a way of yoga.

But it requires a hero *(vìra)* to confront and assimilate, in perfect equanimity, the whole wonder of the World Creatrix—to make love, without hysterical reactions, to the Life-force, which is the sakti of his own entirety. The "five good things" *(Pancatattva)*, which are the "forbidden things" of the ordinary men and women of the herd, serve has sacramental fare for one who not only knows but feels that the World Force *(sakti)* is in essence himself. In Tantra, the worship of the World Creatrix in her own terms is rendered possible; for cohabitation *(maithuna)*, her own supreme holy rite, is realized not in the spirit of the *pasu* ("cattle"; the human animal of the herd, desiring, fearing, and enjoying in the usual animal-human way), but of the *vira* ("hero") who knows himself to be identical with Siva. "Om," he prays (and knows); "into the Fire which is Spirit *(àtman)* brightened by the pouring on of the ghee of merit and demerit, I, by the path of yoga *(susumnà)*, ever sacrifice the functions of the senses, using the mind as the ladle of the offering. Hallelujah !"[32]

The fruit of the rite then is release from illusion, which is the highest gift of Kàlì, the dark and beautiful Goddess-Dancer of the Cremation Ground.

2. The Lamb, the Hero, and the Man-God

"No ONE who is not himself divine may (successfully) worship the divinity (*nàdevo devam arcayet*)."[33] "Having become the deity, one should offer sacrifice to it (*devam bùtvà devam yajet*)."[34] The identity of the hidden nature of the worshiper with the god worshiped is the first principle of the Tàntric philosophy of devotion. The gods are reflexes in space (which is itself the work of màyà-sakti) of that sole reality, Brahman, which is the Sakti of the devotion, the Tàntric sàdhaka approaches the Goddess in worship *(pùjà)*, through the meditative muttering of prayers (*japa:* the recitation of the litany of her names), the unrelenting verbal repetition (again japa*)* of sacred formulae *(mantra:* word-sounds which contain her essence), the making of mental and external offerings *(homa)*, and one-pointed meditation on her inner vision *(dhyàna)*. He could never hope to experience the final identity if he were not already convinced and aware of it from the first. Meanwhile, to support his preliminary approach, he sets before his eyes and mind an image *(Pratìka. Pratima)* of the deity. This may be a statue, painting, symbol of some kind, or yantra;[35] in special cases it may be a living being, for example, a virgin *(kumàrìpùjà)*, or the worshipers's wife.

The first act of devotion consists in contemplating inwardly the mental image of the deity and then projecting the spiritual energy (tejas) of that inner subtle form into the gross outer image. This consecration is known as *prànpratisthà*, "the consignment (*pratisthà*) of the vital breath (*pràna*. "It is to be undone again at the conclusion of the period of worship by a "dismissal" *(visarjana)* of the holy presence, following which the image is no longer the seat of a deity *(pìtha)*, and may be thrown away. The worshiper sends forth and takes back again the shining form, just as the Creator sends forth and takes back again into his infinite substance the manifold of the cosmos- and by virtue of the same infinitude *(brahman-àtman)* within, as well as the same miracle of màyà. Later, when initiate learns to recognize and spontaneously respond to the presence of the divinity everywhere, in all things, he no longer requires the pedagogical assistance of this ritual, but meanwhile his mind and sentimements must be given help. The little miracle of transubstantiation, however, is rather a microcosmic than a macrocosmic crisis. Divinity itself cannot be said to have been actually summoned and dismissed; rather, the *realization* of divinity has been facilitated. For, whereas the adept in the condition of perfect realization beholds and reveres the whole world as an icon or seat *(pìtha)* of the Universal Presence, the usual member of the human herd *(pasu)* requires all the assistance of religion to bring his mind from the common, animal, economic-political mode of considering things, to the contemplative attitude of a luminous intuition.

The rites performed in the presence of a consecrated image are the counterparts of the secular rituals of daily life. The god is welcomed as a guest, with flowers, obeisance, washing of the feet, food, water for bathing, cloth for garments, jewels, perfume, incense, offerings of various kinds, praise, and conversation.[36] These redound, in turn, to the sanctification of daily life; for a guest is welcomed with the same ceremonial; a parent is honoured as a god, and a child attended as a god. The sanctity of the Presence thus perceptibly pervades the social sphere. Ritual gestures *(mudrà)* also are employed in the worship, and these, like words, are the expressions and supports of spiritual resolve. These gestures, or *mudràs*, are identical with those represented in Indian images and utilized in the art of the Indian dance. They constitute a veritable language of the hands, making possible the most subtle amplifications of expression. For example, when presenting, in offering, the vessel of water, the fish gesture *(matsya mudrà)* is made. "This is done as the expression of the wish and intention that the vessel which contains water may be regarded as an ocean with fish and all other aquatic animals. The sadhaka says to the Devata of his worship, 'this is but a small offering of water in fact, but so far as my desire to honour you is concerned, regard it as if I were offering you an ocean.'"[37] Or again, when the Goddess is invited to take her place, before the moment of worship, the *yoni mudra* is made, since the yoni, the female organ, is her pitha or yantra. The yoni can never be regarded by a Tantric adept otherwise than as an altar. Therefore, when the sadhaka has attained to perfection in this discipline he can proceed to the most appropriate and congenial form of paying worship to the Goddess, in maithuna.

Bhùtasuddhi, or "the cleansing *(suddhi)* of the (five) elements of which the body is composed *(bhùta)*," is an indispensable preliminary to every Tantric rite. The devotee imagines the divine power *(sakti)* as being asleep within him, withdrawn from operation in his gross physique, coiled away like a sleeping serpent *(kundalinì)* at the root of his spine, in the deep place known as the *mùlàdhàra*, "the root *(mùla)* base *(àdhàra)*." The sadhaka then pronounces mantra to arouse her, while controlling carefully his inhalations, breathing deeply first through one nostril then the other *(pràṇàyàma)*, to clear the way for her through the spiritual channel *(susumnà)* that is supposed to run through the interior of the spine. He is then to think of her as aroused. She lifts her head and begins to move up the susumna, touching in her passage a number of "centers" or "lotuses" *(cakras, padmas)*, which are regarded as the seats of the elements of the body. The muladhara is the seat of "earth"; it is pictured as a crimson lotus of four petals. The next center above, called *svàdhisthàna* (sakti's "own abode"), is at the level of the genitals and is the seat of the element "water"; it is pictured as a vermilion lotus of six petals. The next, at the level of the navel, is known as *manipùra*, "the city *(pùra)* of the lustrous gem *(mani)*," so called because it is the seat of the element "fire". It is pictured as a blue-black lotus of ten petals. According to the psychology of this system of lotuses: muladhara, svadhisthana, and manipura are the centers from which the lives of most people are governed, while the superior centers represent higher modes of experience. The fourth, at the level of the heart, is the lotus in which the first realization of the divinity of the world is experienced. Here, it is said, the god reaches down to touch his devotee. Or again, here the sages hear the sound *(sabda)* of Brahman. Sounds heard by the outer ear are produced by "two things striking together," whereas the sound of Brahman is *anàhata sabda*, "the sound *(sabda)* which comes without the striking of any two things together *(anàhata)*."[38] This sound is OM; not the OM pronounced by the lips, which is but a mnemonic suggestion produced by the striking of the wind from the lungs upon the organs of the mouth, but the fundamental OM of creation, which is the Goddess herself as sound. Because this is heard in the lotus of the heart, that center is called *anàhata*; it is pictured as a ruddy lotus of twelve petals, and is the seat of the element "air".

"Ether," the fifth and ultimate element, is centered in the cakra of a smoky purple hue and of sixteen petals at the level of the throat. This is the Visuddha Cakra, "the completely purified." Beyond, at the point between the eyebrows, is the Lotus of Command *(àjña)*. White as the moon, possessing two petals, shining with the glory of perfected mediation, wherein the mind, beyond the zones veiled by the five elements and thus completely free of the limitations of the senses, beholds immediately the seed-form of the Vedas. This is the seat of the Form of forms, where the devotee beholds the Lord—as in the Christian heaven. Beyond is the center beyond duality, Sahasrara, the vari coloured lotus of a thousand petals at the crown of the head. Here Sakti—who is to be thought of as having ascended through all the lotuses of the susumnà, waking each lotus to full blossom in passing—is joined to Siva in a union that is simultaneously the fulfillment and dissolution of the worlds of sound, form, and contemplation.

The Tàntric worshiper is supposed to *imagine* himself as having purified his body by suffusing all the lotuses with the awakened Sakti in this way (only a perfected yogi being capable of making the kundalini actually rise). Meditation *((dhyàna)*, the recitation of charms filled with the power of the Goddess in the form of sound *(mantrà)*, eloquent postures of the hands and body *(mudrà)*, and the meditative placing of the tips of the fingers and palm of the right hand on various parts of the body, accompanied by mantra *(nyàsàa,*[39] assist him in this process, as well as in that of welcoming the god into the image or yantra. The two processes are reciprocal, and constitute the whole mystery of ritualistic transubstantiation. Hence we read, in the *Gandharva Tantra*: "A man should worship a divinity *(devatà)* by becoming a divinity himself. One should not worship a divinity without oneself becoming a divinity. If a person worships a divinity without becoming himself a divinity, he will not reap the fruits of that worship."[40] And again, in the *Vàsistha Ràmàyana*: "If a man worships Visnu without himself becoming Visnu, he will not reap the fruits of that worship. If he worships Visnu by becoming himself Visnu, an initiate *(sàdhaka)* will become Great Visnu *(Mahàvisnu,* i.e., the Being that is beyond the personal aspect of the god)."[41] And once again, this time in the *Bhavisya Puràna*: "A man should not mediate on Rudra without himself becoming Rudra,[42] nor take the name of Rudra (by muttering the "garland" of the god's names) without becoming Rudra; nor will he attain Rudra without becoming Rudra."[43]

The act of worship is meant to facilitate a direct, immediate experience of what the sàdhaka already knows theoretically, namely, that jìva and ìsvara (the latter preferably in the feminine form of sakti) are in essence one, being the complementary forms through which Brahman becomes manifest in the field of the pairs-of-opposites, the created world. The sàdhaka confronts his devata, which is represented in the form either of an external image or of an interior vision, on the plane and in the state of dualism, yet he knows that what appears as two is actually one. The activity of self-surrender then leads to the perfect realization of this mystery. Surrender of the illusory sovereignt nature of the individual transforms him into a servant *(dàsa)* of the divinity, and this state, when brought to perfection, then reveals to him his own fundamental sovereignty as the deity itself. The fervor of daily worship through bhakti yoga thus awakens the hidden divine nature in man, and divine ecstatic beatitude *(Prema)* supervenes following the moment of perfect participation. Similarly, the son the wealthy man, in the above-cited parable of the Mahàyàna-Buddhist *Sadharmapundarìka*, without knowing it, served his father as a servant, gradually was advanced in his estate, and eventually came to realize that he was himself the son and heir of the master, entitled to all his possessions; indeed, himself the rich man, the alter-ego of his lord.[44]

But the rites and grades of service are governed by the spiritual character of the devotee. This is a basic principle of all Indian psychological training. The personality endowed with rajas (the quality of vigor and action) will require a different sadhana from one steeped in tamas, while the godlike man of brilliant sattva will be fit for still another way. In the Tantric vocabulary these three types are known, respectively, as *vìra*, the hero, *pasu*, the dark-witted animal of the herd, and *divya*, the godlike, luminous saint.

It is noteworthy, and perhaps a symptom of Ksatriya provenience, that in the classic Tàntric Àgamas the emphasis is given to the vira, the man of ràjasic disposition. According to the ideal and way of the Vedànta, rajas was to be subdued by sattva, all the disciplines being founded on the principle of the perfect mirror-pond, but in the classic Tàntric realization the victory was achieved by way of the passions themselves: they were challenged, directly faced, and ridden as a mettlesome stallion by a knight. The "five good things," which for the pasu, the pedestrian, the man of the herd, represent only danger, became the pre eminent vehicles of attainment. "The five essential elements in the worship of Sakti," the *Mahànirvàna Tantra* states, "have been prescribed to be wine, meat, fish, parched grain, and the union of man with woman. The worship of Sakti without these five elements is but the practice of evil magic (*abhicàra*: a ritual that injures or destroys); the power that is the object of the discipline is never attained thereby, and obstacles are encountered at every step. As seed sown on barren rocks does not germinate, so worship *(Pùjà)* without these five elements is fruitless."[45] These statements are quoted in the text as the words of Siva to his Sakti, pronounced in the inner chamber of their divinely blissful abode, on the summit of the sacred mountain Kailàsa.

Neither the saintly nor the gentlemanly Hindu of today, however, favors the boldness of this heroic view. Instead, the attitude formerly assigned to the Pasu is recommended for all, that namely of worshiping the life force *(sakti)* not as the Bride but as the Mother, and thus submitting, like a child, to a sort of sacramental castration. "The attitude of a 'hero,'" said Ràmakrishna to one of the most worldly of his devotees, Girish Chandra Ghosh, a successful dramatist and the director of the Calcutta "Star Theatre": "The attitude of a, 'hero' is not good. Some people cherish it. They regard themselves as Purusa and woman as Prakrti; they want to propitiate woman through their intercourse with her. But this method often causes disaster."

GIRISH: "At one time I too cherished that idea."

Sri Ramakrishna gazed at Girish pensively, in silence.

GIRISH: "I still have that twist in my mind. Tell me what I should do."

RÀMAKRISHNA *(following a moment of silent consideration)*: "Give God your power of attorney. Let Him do whatever He likes."

Abruptly, the conversation was then turned to a discussion of Ramakrishna's younger devotees.

RÀMAKRISHNA *(to Girish and the rest)*: "In meditation I see the inner traits of these youngsters. They have no thought of acquiring house and property. They do not crave sex pleasure. Those of the youngsters who are married do not sleep with their wives. The truth is that unless a man has gor rid of rajas and has acquired sattva, he cannot steadily dwell in God; he cannot love God and realize Him."

GIRISH: "You have blessed me."

RÀMAKRISHNA: "How is that ? I said that you would succeed if you were sincere."

Before Girish could respond, Srì Ràmakrishna cried, with a shout of joy, "Ànandamayì !" and the company saw him—as they had beheld him many times before—pass abruptly from normal consciousness to the trance state of divine absorption *(samàdhì)*. He remained abstracted for some time, but presently moved, and soon was back again, vivaciously participating in the conversation.[46]

One of his "youngsters" had inquired, on a former occasion: "Isn't it true that the Tantra prescribes spiritual discipline in the company of women ?"

"That," the Master had replied, "is not desirable. It is a very difficult path and often causes the aspirant's downfall. There are three such kinds of discipline. One may regard woman as one's mistress or look on oneself as her handmaid, or as her child. I look on woman as my mother. To look on oneself as her handmaid is also good; but it is extremely difficult to practice spiritual discipline looking on woman as one's mistress. To regard oneself as her child is a very pure attitude."[47]

And on another occasion: "Sakti alone is the root of the universe. That Primal Energy has two aspects: vidyà and avidyà. Avidyà deludes. Avidyà conjures up 'woman and gold,' which casts the spell. Vidyà begets devotion, kindness, wisdom, and love, which lead one to God. This avidya must be propitiated, and that is the purpose of thierties of Sakti worship.

"The devotee assumes various attitudes toward Sakti in order to propitiate Her: the attitude of a handmaid, a 'hero,' or a child. A hero's attitude is to please Her even as a man pleases a woman through intercourse.

"The worship of Sakti is extremely difficult. It is no joke. I passed two years as the handmind and companion of the Divine Mother. But my natural attitude has always been that of a child toward its mother. I regard the breasts of any woman as those of my own mother. Woman are, all of them, the veritable images of Sakti."[48]

In the classic Tàntric Àgamas three varieties of sàdhanà are prescribed for the various temperaments. That of the "five good things," as we have described them, is for the vira. But for the pasu, these are still the "five for bidden things." And so the term "wine" *(madya)* is interpreted in his case to mean coconut water, milk, or some other indicated "substitutional substance" *(anukalpatattva)*. Similarly, instead of "meat" *(màmsa)*, he partakes of wheat-beans, ginger, sesamum, salt, or garlic, and instead of "fish" *(mastya)*, for red radish, red sesamum, masur (a kind of grain), the white brinjal vegetable, and paniphala (an aquatic plant). "Parched grain" *(mudrà)* in the form of rice, wheat, paddy, etc., is permitted, but instead of maithuna, childlike submission is recommended before the Divine Mother's Lotus Feet.[49]

The divya, the god-man of purest sattva, on the other hand, is far, far beyond both the "substitutional," safe-and-sane sàdhana of the pious lamb, but also beyond the fearless, chivalric experiences of the hero. For him no external image or sacrament whatsoever is required. Hence, in the rereading of the "five good things" as prescribed for the divya, "`wine' *(madya)* is not any liquid, but that intoxicating knowledge acquired by yoga of the Parabrahman which renders the worshiper senseless as regards the external world. `Meat' *(màmsa)* is not any fleshly thing, but the act whereby the sadhaka consigns all his acts to `Me' *(mm)*, that is, the Lord (this, of course, is a pun). `Fish' *(matsya)* is that sattvic knowledge by which through the sense of `mineness' ( a play upon the word *matsya*) the worshiper sympathizes with the pleasure and pain of all beings. *Mudrà* is the act of relinquishing all association with evil which results in bondage. While `coition' *(maithuna)* is the union of the Sakti Kundalinì, the `Inner woman' and World-force in the lowest center *(mùlàdhàra cakra)* of the sadhaka's own body with the supreme Siva in the highest center *(sahasràra)* in his upper brain.[50]

For, whereas the pasu or vìra devotee practicing bhùtasuddhi (the ritual purification of the elements of the body in preparation for an act of dualistic worship)[51] has to *imagine* the purifying ascent of the Kundalinì through the centers or lotuses *(cakras, padmas)* of the susumna, the divya, adept in the exercises of the Tàntric Kundalinì Yoga, actually brings this psychosomatic miracle to pass. Àsana and mudrà (proper seat and posture), prànàyàma (control of the breath), dhyàna and mantrà (interior visualization and the concentrated recitation of certain "seed" sounds and formulae), following a long and severe preliminary training in physical and emotional self-purification, lead actually to a physical effect which is described as the channeling of all the energies of the body into a subtle channel up the interior of the spine *(susumna)*. In this case, the rise of the "serpent Power" *(kundalinì)* and awakening of the lotuses *(padmas)* does not have to be imagined, it actually comes to pass. And when the sixth center is attained—the "Lotus of Command" *(àjñà)* between the eyebrows—the Lord *(ìsvara)* is actually seen, not simply imagined, and the beholder is completely lost in savikalpa sàmadhi—communion with the Brahman "with limitations" *(savikalpa)*, where the distinction between the subject and the personal God is retained.[52] Whereas the moment the rising force then enters the ultimate thousand-petalled lotus at the crown of the head (the sahasràra), where Siva and Sakti are one, the knowledge of duality is in sheer experience transcended, and the state of the yogì becomes that of nirvikalpa samadhi: realization of the identity of Àtman with the Brahman "beyond all limitations" *(nirvikalpa)*, where both the subject and its highest object are annihilate.[53]

"There is one simple test whether the Sakti (= *kundalinì*) is actually aroused," writes Sir John Woodroffe. "When she is aroused intense heat is felt at that spot, but when she leaves a particular center the part so left becomes as cold and apparently lifeless as a corpse. The progress upwards may thus be externally verified by others. When the Sakti (Power) has reached the upper brain *(sahasràra)* the whole body is cold and corpselike; except the top of the skull, where some warmth is felt, this being the place where the static and kinetic aspects of Consciousness unite."[54]

"Sometimes the Spiritual current rises through the spine, crawling like an ant," Ràmakrishna told a circle of his intimate friends. "Sometimes, in samàdhi, the soul swims joyfully in the ocean of divine ecstasy, like a fish. Sometimes, when I lie down on my side, I feel the Spiritual current pushing me like a monkey and playing with me joyfully, I remains still. That current. like a monkey, suddenly with one jump reaches the Sahasrara. That is why you see me jump up with a start.

"Sometimes, again, the Spiritual Current rises like a bird hopping from one branch to another. The place where it rests feels like fire. It may hop from Mùlàdhàra to svàdhisthàna, from Svàdhisthàna to the heart, and thus gradually to the head. Sometimes the spiritual Current moves up like a snake. Going in a zigzag way, at last it reaches the head and I go into samàdhi.

"A man's spiritual consciousness is not awakened unless his Kundalini is aroused. The Kundalinì dwells in the Mùlàdhàra. When it is aroused, it passes along the Susumna nerve, goes through the centers of Svàdisthàna, Manipùra, and so on, and at last reaches the head. This is called the movement of the Mahavayu, the Spiritual Current. It culminates in samadhi.

"One's spiritual consciousness is not awakened by the mere reading of books. One should pray to God. The Kundalini is aroused if the aspirant feels restless for God. To talk of knowledge from mere study and hearsay ! What will that accomplish ?

"Just before my attaining this state of mind, it had been revealed to me how the Kundalilnì is aroused, how the lotuses of the different centers blossom forth, and how all this culminates in samàdhi. This is a very secret experience. I saw a boy twenty-two or twenty-three years old, exactly resembling me, enter the Susumnà nerve and commune with the lotuses, touching them with his tongue. He began with the center at the a minus and passed through the centers of the sexual organs, navel, and so on. The different lotuses of those centers—four-petalled, six petalled, and so forth—had been drooping. At his touch they stood erect.

"When he reached the heart—I distinctly remember it—and communed with the lotus there, touching it with his tongue, the twelve-petalled lotus, which was hanging head down, stood erect and opened its Petals. Then he came to the sixteen-petalled lotus in the throat and the two-petalled lotus in the throat and the two-petalled lotus in the forehead. And last of all, the

thousand-petalled lotus in the head blossomed. Since then I have been in this state,"*

"Waken, O Mother!" wrote Ramprasad, "O Kundalinì, whose nature is Bliss Eternal! Thou art the serpent coiled in sleep, in the lotus of the Muladhara!"[56]

"In dense darkness, O Mother," runs another wonderful song, "Thy formless beauty sparkles":

In dense darkness, O Mother, Thy formless beauty sparkles;
Therefore the yogis meditate in a dark mountain cave.

In the lap of boundless dark, on Mahànirvàna's waves upborne,
Peace flows serene and inexhaustible.

Taking the form of the Void, in the robe of darkness wrapped,

Who art Thou, Mother, seated alone in the shrine of samàdhi ? From the Lotus of Thy fear-scattering Feet flash Thy love's lightening;

Thy Spirit-Face shines forth with laughter terrible and loud.[57]

3. All the Gods within Us

IN THE Jaina and kindred teachings, matter is described as of an inert and lifeless *(ajìva)* character. The ruthless asceticism of the "naked philosophers" (the "gymnosophists" who astounded Alexander's Greeks) followed logically from their resolution to be sterilized of this dead material and thus rendered pristine—pure, luminous, and perfect. Like balloons leaving the earth below—the earth, its atmosphere, and even the ultimate stratospheric envelope—their life-monads were leaving beneath them, trait by trait, the universal bandages of lifeless "life" As we have seen, the force in India of that pre-Àryan, dualistic, yogic point of view was so great that even the exuberant monism of the Bràhmans finally submitted to its life-searing influence. Gradually, the vigorous world-affirmation of the Vedic period underwent a strangely contradictory change, until, in what is generally regarded as the supreme nondualistic designation of Brahman as *sat, cit, ànanda* ("pure being, consciousnes, and bliss," absolutely uninvolved in the bondage, ignorance, and misery of the world illusion) the yogic principle won its most impressive triumph. For although it is true that instead of the pre-Àryan, jaina, and Yoga ideal of the "isolation-integration" *(kaivalya)* of separate life-monads *(jìvas, purusas)* the new goal was that of reunion with the one Saccidànanda Brahman, "one-without-a-second," nevertheless this nondual reunion, this recognition of an identity which in reality had never been forfeited, was understood as being synonymous with a refutation of the false notion of the existence of a cosmos: a dissolution of the "superimposition" due to "ignorance". "That which is untouched by the sixfold wave [of decay and death, hunger and thirst, grief and delusion], meditated upon by the yogi's heart but not grasped by the sense-organs, which the faculty of intuition *(buddhi)* cannot know, and which is faultless *(anavadyam)*: that Brahman art thou—meditate upon this in thy mind."[58] The same, basic ascetic attitude of rejection as that which in the pre-

Àryan past has sundered human experience into the spheres of ajìva and jìva, was now discriminating between samsàra and nirvana, while striving for identification ("without remainder") with the unimplicated term.

And yet, on the other hand, ther flourishes in India, side by side with this attitude of negation, a vigorous affirmation of the world of flux and time, which is just as fearless and absolute, in its own way, as the unflinching self-transcendence of the yogis. In that land the great human effort, looking either way, seems always to have been to break the all-too-human limitations of the mind by means of "inhuman" techniques. The ideals and disciplines of the castes are "inhuman"—humanistically speaking; and in a sense, every Indian, one way or another, is a yogi: for bhakti, the popular Hindu "path of devotion," is itself yoga: an internal "yoking" of the mind to a divine principle. Wherever bhakti is carried to an ultimate statement, as for instance in the *Bhagavad Gìta* and the sacraments of the Tàntric "five good things" *(pañcatattva)*, the secular initiate is inspired to a challenge and assimilation of the *immanent* aspect of absolute Being, which is no less audacious than the corresponding effort, in the penitential groves, to assimilate the *transcendent*.

The Bràhman mind, in other words, did not capitulate unconditionally to the principle of world-rejection. The psychophysical problems posed by the Vedic monist philosophy that matured during the period of the Upanisads are as open to world-assertive as to negating replies. The more amply documented Indian philosophical tendency, and the one first encountered by the Western scholars, was that represented in the schools of the Vedànta and Hìnayàna, but in recent years the power and profundity of the Tàntric system have begun to be appreciated, and therewith has been facilitated a new understanding of Indian life and art. Indeed, one could only have been amazed had it been found that in the most durable civilization known to history the sole intellectual response to such a dictum as "All Is Brahman" had ben that of a monastic renunciation of the manifest for the unmanifest aspect of the metaphysical equation. Had we not learned what we now know of the philosophy of the Tàntric Agàmas; we should have had to posit some such tradition;

for as the Indian centuries open their secrets to us we become more and more aware of the power of something very different from the sublimated melancholy of the monks, in the life-loving Hindu contemplation of the delicacies of the world of name and form. In the majestic sculptural rendering of Siva Trimùrti at Elephanta,[59] in the now well-known South-Indian bronzes of the Dancing Siva,[60] in the phantasmagoric "foam and mist" style of the great masterpieces of Bhàjà, Màmallapuram, and Elùrà,[61] as well as in the Indian aesthetic phenomenon which I have elsewhere described as that of "expanding form,"[62] a stupendous dionysian affirmation of the dynamism of the phenomenal spectacle is rendered, which at once affirms and transcends the apprehended traits of the individual and his cosmos. Prakrti herself (*natura naturans*, not the merely visible surface of things) is here portrayed—with no resistance to her charm—as She gives birth to the oceans of the worlds. Individuals—mere waves, mere moments, in the rapidly flowing, unending torrent of ephemeral forms —are tangibly present; but their tangibility itself is simply a gesture, an affectionate flash of expression on the otherwise invisible countenance of the Goddess Mother whose play *(lìlà)* is the universe of her own beauty. In this dionysian vision the individual is at once devaluated and rendered divine, majectic with the majesty of Nature herself and mystically sheltered in the very maelstrom of the world.

Such a view, obviously, is not fit for all. It can appeal to only certain types and tastes: the aristocratic, for example, or the artistic, and the ecstatic. An intellectual temperament , though perhaps appreciative of the torrential magnitude of such a vision, will remain, necessarily, somewhat cool, refusing to respond to it with the whole personality. That is why this view—though certainly perennial in India—is less well documented in literature, theology, and philosophy than in the works of art. The texts are from the hands of intellectuals, by nature endowed for the abstract realizations of the way of disembodied thought *(jñàna-yoga);* but the art works have poured from the hands of craftsmen commissioned by wealthy merchants and aristocrats—all the children, the servants, or the willing heroes of the Goddess; perhaps profoundly respectful of her more thoughtful sons, yet intimately aware, all the time, that there are riches, boons, and wondrous paradoxical insights that She holds in store only for those who truly dote on Her, and which the haughty discriminators, dedicated to the transcendental One-without-a-second, can never share.

Throughout the known history of India these two points of view have operated in a dialectic process of antagonistic cooperation to bring to pass the majestic evolution of art, philosophy, ritual and religion, political, social, economic, and literary forms, which we know today as the miracle of Indian civilization. By and large, it can be said that the nondual world-affirmation of the Vedic Bràhmans, with its wider swing and greater depth, has been the dominant and victorious contributor to the development. To the pluralistic-realistic, idealistic dualism of jaina-Sankhya stamp we can ascribe only a preliminary and provocative role. By virtue of a blood and vigours technique of philosophizing in paradoxes, continually establishing the essential unity of terms and spheres that would logically appear to be antagonistic. the fertile thought of Bràhmanism unfailingly brought together. fused, and transcended the pairs-of-opposites, which were then allowed to proceed again from each other in a brilliant dialectical play; Brahmanic thought being the philosophic counterpart and expression of the life-process itself, a reflection in conceptual terms of the paradoxology of life's unceasing dynamism.

Food, flesh, and blood become transformed in a living body into impulses, emotions, feelings, thought, and inspiration. These in turn condition and move the bodily frame. Then the decomposition of the same body after death converts it into the teeming life of worms and vegetation, which again is food. There is a continuous circuit of metabolism, an unending transformation of opposites into each other. And this reality of becoming is what is mirrored in the Bràhmanic monist conception of màyà. The perpetual motion of things turning into each other is the reality denoted by the icon of the Goddess. The female conceives by the male and transforms his seed into their common offspring, a new formation of their substance. Such is the miracle of the enigma, Màyà-Sakti. Hers, therefore, is an erotic life-philosophy, precisely the opposite and exact compliment of the sterilizing, stern, sublime, ascetic thinking of the Jaina-Sankhya schools.

The concern of the latter is to divide, to cleanse of each other, and finally to separate forever, the life-principle, which is incorporeal, and the principle of both gross and subtle matter, which is life-conditioning, life-staining and -obscuring. In the long course of Indian thought, this stern ascetic attitude has been able to celebrate its moments of victory, and these moments have contributed immeasurably to the recolouring and renovation of Indian life. But that life itself, in accordance with its own innate dialectic principle of transformation, has then inevitably brought to pass a new miracle of absorption, assimilation, and restatement: time and time again, great, vigorous, tropical India has adopted the sublime way of sterilization, the way supremely represented in the teachings of the Buddha and in Sankara's Vedanta; but always the powers and wisdom of the erotic-paradoxical monism of life—and of the Brahman understanding—has again successfully reasserted its force.

Brahman, sakti, the force-substance of Indian nondual philosophy, is the principle that enters, pervades, and animates the panorama and evolutions of nature, but as the same time is the animated and pervaded, entered field or matter of nature itself *(prakrti, natura naturans)*; thus it both *inhabits* and *is* the manifested universe and all its forms. As the unceasing dynamism of the transitory sphere of becoming and withering away, it lives in all the changes of birth, growth, and dissolution.

But, simultaneously, it is remote from this sphere of change; for in its quiescent, dormant transcendent aspect it knows no phases and is detached form both the living and the dead. The names ascribed to it are concessions to the human mind. This mind, however, being itself of the essence of the unutterable, may be touched to Self-recollection by properly hearing one or another of the finally inadequate names. The name Brahman, Saccidànanda Brahman, is misleading; for it suggests that the transcendent *is*. The name Vacuity, Sùnyatà, the Void, is misleading also; for it suggests that the transcendent *is not*. Perhaps, though, the latter is the less misleading and therefore the better term; for it does suggest transcendence, rather than definable existence. Nevertheless, the difference is not seriously worth an argument. As a clue either term will serve, whereas if not properly understood neither means a thing.

Bràhman philosophy produced its last synthesizing statement in the courageous esotericism of the Tantras and in the Tàntric Mahàyàna (the latter surviving today in the snow-clad summits and high dales of Tibet), where the old Àryan frenzy for non-dualism and the paradox, forever asserting the unity of incompatibles, fruitfully combined with its own incompatible—the archaic matrilineal world-feeling of the aboriginal civilization of India. What the Vedic sages had recognized in the heavens of the macrocosm, the Tàntric adept felt dwelling bodily within himself, in the microcosm, and he named it, also, "God." Hence, whereas the members of the Bràhman caste in Vedic times had conjured the holy power *(brahman)* by means of public sacrifices, the Tàntric devotee, of whatever caste, by means of the simple, essentially personal rituals of the circles of Tàntric initiates, sacrificed his own ego and thereby conjured the holy power *(Sakti)* of his own phenomenality into manifestation in his life. The goods served by the Bràhmans had been those of the community; the god worshiped by the Tantrist was his own, his *ista-devatà*, his chosen beloved—which yet was identical in essence with whatever deity was anywhere adored; for "It is only a food, "states the *Sammohana Tàntra*, "Who sees any difference between Ràma and Siva."[63] The eligibility of the Bràhman to serve and conjure the gods of the community had rested in the high rank of his caste in that community, whereas the eligibility of the Tàntric devotee reposed in the ripeness of his mind and power of experience. "The Bràhman who is a descendent of a Rsi, or holy sage," we read in the *Satapatha Bràhmana*, "is all the gods."[64] "I am the Devi and none other," thinks the Tantric devotee. "I am Bràhman who is beyond all grief. I am a form of Saccidànanda whose true nature is eternal Liberation."[65]

The idea of the godhood of the individual is thus democratized in the Tantra, because understood psychologically instead of sociopolitically. As a result, the entire context of the public Indian faith has been reinterpreted. The rites and religiosity of contemporary India exhibit in every trait the profound influence of this Tàntric view; indeed, they have ben for centuries more Tàntric than Vedic. In spite of vestigial remains of the archaic snobbism of caste, native Indian life is shot through with the radiance of a realization of universal divinity. In contrast to the attitude of Job who cried out to Yahweh: "What is man, that thou shouldest magnify him ?" the Indian, by shattering his ego, equates himself with God, transcends God, transcends God, and is at peace in the knowledge of himself with God, transcends God, and is at peace in the knowledge of himself with God, transcends God, and is at peace in the knowledge of himself as Brahman. "The Mother is present in every house," writes Ramprasad. "Need I break the news as one breaks an earthen pot on the floor ?"

FOOTNOTE

1 *Supra*, pp. 534.535.

2 *The Gospel of Srì Ràmakrishna*, translated with an introduce by Swami Nikhilananda, New York, 1942, p. 858.

3 *Ib.*, p. 288.

4 Contrast *supra*, p. 439.

5 Brahman as Being *(sat)*, Consciousnes *(cit)*, and Bliss *(ànada)*. Cf. *supra*, p. 425.

6 *The Gospel of Srì Ràmakrishna*, pp. 345-346.

7 Known as màyà the Vedànta; cf. *supra*, pp. 425-427. Sakti is Yum of the Yab-Yum icon; cf. *supra*, pp. 556-559.

8 This idea of the play *(lìlà)* of the Godhead in the forms of the world is fundamental to the Tàntric view and is the Hindu counterpart of the Mahàyàna-Buddhist Mahàsukha (*supra*, p. 554).

9 *The Gospel of Srì Ràmakrishna*, pp. 133-135.

10 For an account of the ideals and history of the Brahmo Samaj (founded in 1828 by Ràjà Rammohan Roy), see Swàmì Nikhilananda's introduction to *The Gospel of Sri Rama-krishna*, pp. 40-42. A distinguished figure in the movement was Devendranath Tagore (1817-1905), father of the Nobel Prize poet, Sir Rabindranath (1861-1941).

11 *Ib.*, pp. 135-139 (with a few brief omissions).

12 The Àgamas (Tàntric writings) are divided into five main groups according to the personification celebrated: Sùrya (the sun god), Ganesa ("Lord of the Hosts," the elephant-headed son of Siva, who is the Indian counterpart of Hermes, breaker of the way and guide of the sul), Sakti, Siva, and Visnu, lathe last three being today by far the most important. Tàntric principles and practices have been applied also to the worship of the Mahàyàna Buddhas and Bodhisattvas; the Yab-Yum symbolism is Tàntric.

13 For a discussion both of this development and of the symbolism of the Goddess, cf. Zimmer, *Myths and Symbols in Indian Art and Civilization* p. 90-102 and 189ff; also *The King and the Corpse* Part II, "The Romance of the Goddess."

14 *The Gospel of Sri Ràmkrishna*, p. 116.

15 *Kularanava Tantra*, cited by Sir John Woodroffe, *Shakti and Shakta*, 3rd edition, Madras and London, 1929, p.7.

16 *Ib.*, p.8. For the term *sàstra* cf. *supra*, p. 36.

17 Dinesh Chandra Sen, *History of Bengali Language and Literature*, Calcutta, 1911, p. 714.

18 *supra*, p.l 561; cf. E. J. Thompson, "A Poet of the People," *The*

London Quarterly Review, CXXX, Fifth Series, XVI (July-October, 1918), p. 71.

19 *The Gospel of Srì Ràmakrishna*, p. 139.

20 Cf. *supra*, p. 41.

21 *The Gospell of sri Ràmakrishna,* p.139.

22 Mudrà also denotes the mystic hand postures that play such an important role in Indian ritual and art. This is the only meaning of the word given in the Sanskrit dictionaries. We read, however, in the *Yogini Tantra* (Ch. VI): "Fried paddy and the like—in fact all such [cereals] as are chewed—are called Mudrà" (cited by Woodroffe, op. cit., p. 571).

23 Cf. Supra, pp. 554-5559.

24 *Gandharva Tantra* 2; Woodroffe, op. cit., p. 538.

25 *Yoginì Tantra* 1; Woodfoffe, op. cit., p. 493.

25 For the term *àsrama,* cf. *supra,* pp. 155-160.

26 *Taittirrìya Bràhmana* 2. 8.8; cf. *supra*, pp. 345-347.

27 Cf. *supra*, pp. 447-455.

28 Cf. *supra*, p. 52.

29. Cf. *supra*, p. 459.

30. Cited by Woodroffe, op. cit., p. 593.

31. Woodroffe, op. cit., pp.l 587-588.

32. Om *Dharmàdharma-havirdìpte àtmàgnan manasà srucà Susumnàvartmanànityam aksvrttìr juhomyaham: Svàhà. (Tantraasàra 698;* Woodroffe, op. cit., p. 559.)

33. Cf. Arthur Avalon (Sir John Woodroffe). *The serpent pow*er 3rd revised edition, Mardras and London, 1931, p.120.

34. An example of *nyàsa* in Christian worship is the making of the sign of the cross, touching first the forehead ("in the name of the Father"), then the breast ("and of the Son"), the left shoulder ("and of the Holy."), right shoulder ("Ghost"), and finally bringing the palms together in the position of salutation known to the Hindus as *añjali*, which is the classic Christian mudra of prayer ("Amen").

The authors of *The Principles of Tantra* (edited by Arthur Avalon, 2 vols., London, 1914-1916), have aptly cited (pp. Ixxi-lxxii) the following statement from the Council of Trent: "The Catholic Church, rich with the experience of the ages and clothed with their spend or, has introduced mystic benediction *(mantra)*, incise *(dhùpa)*, water *(àcamana, padya*, etc.), lights *(dìpa)*, bells *(ghantà)*, flowers *(puspa)*, vestments, and all the magnificence of its ceremonies in order to excite the spirit of religion to the contemplation of the profound mysteries which they reveal. As are its faithful, the Church is composed of both body *(deha)* and soul *(atman)*.

It therefore renders to the Lord *(ìsvara)* a double worship, exterior *(vàhya-pùjà)* and interior *(mànasa-pùjà)*, the latter being the prayer *f (vadana)* of the faithful, the breviary of its priest, and the voice of Him ever interceding in our fever, and the former the outward motions of the liturgy." (Interpolations by authors of *The Principles of Tantra.)*

As to the historical relationship of the Christian to the Tantric service, that is a delicate matter yet to be investigated.

35. Cited by Arthur Avalon, *The Great Liberation*, Madras, 1927, p. 109, note.

36. Vàsìstha Ràmàyana (*Yoga-vasistha*, cited ib.).

37 Rudra is the violent, world-destructive aspect of Siva.

38 *Bhavisya Puràna.* (Avalon cites, in *The Great Liberation* somewhat closely, *Agni Purana.*).

41 Saddharma-pundrìka 4; cf. *supra*, pp. 508-509.

42 *Mahànirvàna Tantra* 5. 22-24. (Translation by Avalon, *The Great Liberation*, pp. 89-90).

43 *The Gospel of Srì Ràmakrishna*, p. 682.

44 *Ib.*, p. 123.

45 *Ib.*, p. 116.

46 Woodroffe, *Shakti and Shàkta*, pp. 569-570.

47 Nilamani Mukhyopadhyaya, *Pancatattva-vicara*, p. 85: Woodroffe, *Shakti and Shàkta*, p. 567. Other sublimated readings of the pañcatatva apear in other texts; cf. Woodroffe, pp. 495-500, 568-569.

48 Cf. *supra*, pp. 584-585.

49 Cf. *supra*, pp. 435-436.

50 Cf. *supra*, pp. 436-437.

51 Avalon, *The Serpent Power*, pp. 21-22.

52 *The Gosspel of Srì Ràmakrishna*, pp. 829-830.

53 *Ib.*, p. 363.

54 *Ib.*, p. 692.

55 Sankara, *Vivekacudàmani* 256.

56 Cf. Zimmer, *Myths and Symbols in Indian Art and Civilization*, pp. 148-151, and fig. 33.

57 *Ib.*, pp. 151-175, and fig. 38.

58 *Ib.*, pp. 53-54, 117-121, 187-188, and figs. 1, 27, 28, 55, 59, and 60.

59 *Ib.*, pp. 130-136.

60 *Sammohana Tantra* 9; Woodroffe, *Shakti and Shàkta*, p. 53.

61 *Satapatha Bràhmana* 12. 4. 4. 6.

62 Woodroffe, *Shakti and Shàkta*, p. 81.

CHAPTER - 4

Applied side of Tantra: Dance, Music, Astrology, Sarcraments

CHAPTER - 4

1. Introduction:

Application of any principle is one of the deciding factors of its scundness. For instance, in the realm of science, the law of gravitation is considered as an authentic or universal law. The reason of it is that it deals unexceptionally with all objects of the universe. Whatever we throw upward necessarily comes downward. In addition to this type of instance, we may add the law of causation which states that every effect presupposes a cause, or in other words, cause necessarily creates effect. All these laws are universal and their application decides the soundness of that branch of knowledge from which they emanate. Being a system, Tantra is also based on some principles among them the cardinal ore is the principle of cultivating of energy. Significance of energy in life needs no illustration. Life or energy is the core of universe. Tantra has found out the source of energy, not only that, but it has also mentioned the way of cultivation and channelization of it.

For Tantra, energy is the Ultimate Reality. Everthing is but its manifestation. It creates, sustains and destroys. How does it this work ? Energy does this through vibration and movement which are its unavoidable aspects. So these two also can be the aids of the realization of energy. Indian arts like of Music and Dance are based on these two aspects respectively.

The root of the term Nratya is I nruta means "to act" which is highly related with movements. A dancer through different gestures (Mudràs) or movements creates his/her own universe on the stage. Through the rhythmical movements he/she is attuned to the entire cosmic movements. In this way he/she establishes an identity of the finite with infinite which is our goal.

Like dance, music also ends into realizsation. In music, notes (svara) enjoy significant status. In Tantra, these svara are considered as the Nàda sakti or cosmic, sound which is one of the aspects of the Kundalinì sakti, the universal power. As in Vedos, so in Tantra also, Sabda is considered as Brahman or energy. Being a manifestation of the Nàda sakti, each and every letter is highly powerful. This power is felt through the medium of vibration. And because of this we feel the impact of the arranged Raga of music.

Each and every atom of the universe, being a manifestation of energy, issues vibrations. We are not the only entity in the universe but there is a wide planetary system also. This also, like us, constantly issues electric currents. According to the Tàntric principle of identity between microcosm and macrocosm, attraction and repulsion takes place which becomes the deciding factor of the favourable and unfavourable impact of the planetary system. Harmony between vibrations of the subject and planets give favour while disharmony gives unfavour. The Indian astrology is based on this Tàntric principle.

Apparently this leads us to conclude that we are slave of the planetary system. But according to Tantra, it is not so. Our mind is more powerful than planetary system. Power is there but it is latent in mind. A siddha or an expert can compel the planetary system through his cultivated mental powers.

The primitive man believed that the cause of pleasure and pain is the super natural power. For the benign influence on the important occasions of life which start from conception to cremation ground which are sixteen in number (Sodasa Samskàra) are still being celebrated with the help of Mantras and Yantras.

Like above mentioned aspects, the influence of Tàntric principles are also discernible on other aspects of life but within the limit of this is, we shall see something about the above mentioned aspects. We shall proceed with the dance-an expression of innate creative energy.

A. Dance:

For Tantra, energy is the Ultimate Reality of which constant movement is the unavoidable aspect. Tàntric Lord Siva is considered as the lord of dance, Nrityamurti or Natraja-a master dancer.

Rhythm both in universe and in dance also is unavoidable aspect. In universe, we see the process of creation, maintenance and destruction in a rhythmical order being constantly done by cosmic Reality. Beyond these there are also two aspects which are namely, grace (Anugraha) and concealment (Tirdhdhàna). These five fold aspect of Reality is symbolized in a posture of Natraja , the great dancer.

The dancing posture of hands and legs of Natràja is not also out of significance. This posture suggests Siva as most beneficial to mankind. The right hand with drum and fire symbolizes the hand of protection (Abhaya) while left hand with dandam is a hand of bestowing the boons. This is the description of the exoteric form of posture Natràja. Now let us see what it esoterically represents.

(i) *Esoteric meaning of the dancing posture of Siva :*

The esoteric significance of the posture Natràja suggests the Tàntric principle of identity between microcosm and macrocosm or Individual self and the Universal self. As the universe is the stage of cidambram of Lord Siva on which He dances, the same cidambaram is located in the body, that is, his heart where God's image eternally dances for destroying the Mayà and release the spirit within. As Rao Gopinath has rightly observed, "Siva is a destroyer and loves the burning ground. But what does He destroy ? Not merely the heavens and earth at the end of a kalpa, but the fetters that bind each separate soul. Where and what is the burning ground. It is not the place where our earthly bodies are cremated, but the heart of the bhakta, the devotee laid waste and disolate. He brings not peace but a sword. The place where their selves are destroyed signifies the place or state where their ego, or illusion and deeds are brunt away: that is the crematorium, the burning ground where Sri Natraja dances. I

Siva as destroyer is known as Mahàkàla who even in the work of destruction, constantly creates. The consort of Siva as Mahakala is known as 'Tandava'. Either way it is the movement of energy that brings about change in the cosmos. Now let us see something about the dance of Kàli.

(ii) *Dance of Kàli or energy: Làsya Nritya :*

We have got glimpse of Siva as lord of dance. Through His dance, He does five fold activities namely, creation, maintenance, destruction, grace and concealment. He does this with the help of his consort, Sakti Kàli, who inspires Siva to express any gesture.

Sakti is also a dancer. She dances on the prostrate body of her lover, Siva. This posture is also highly significant. Sir John Woodroffe has beautifully disclosed the significance of the dancing posture of Kàli, or energy. In his own words, "She is naked being clothed in space alone (Digambara) because Great power is unlimited; further she is Herself beyond `Màyà' that power of Herself with which she creates all universe. She stands upon the white corpse like body of Siva. He is white because He is the illumination. (Prakàsha), the transcendental aspect of consciousness. He is inert because He is the changeless aspect of the Supreme and She is apparently the changing aspect of the same, being twin aspects of the one who is changeless and exists as change."[2]

Tantric principles are not related only with the esoteric meaning of dance. But its technique, like the Hathoyogic postures (àsanàs), pranayama are also connected with the gesturers (Mudras) of dance.

(iii) *Dance and Hathayogic technique :*

Dance is not merely a movement of body but it also represents the exposition of the moods and emotions of mind. For perfect presentation of moods, mind should be calm and this calmness can be gained through prànàyàma. Like calmness, the flexibility of body is also required in dance. The Hatha yogic asanas secure this. So with the help of àsanàs and prànayàma, a dancer can express his/ her emotions perfectly.

The above mentioned fact is realized by Zdena Bronislaw Ska Deylova. Her experience has been published in the "Yoga" journal of April, 1978, in which she has accepted that the practice of the Hathayogic asanas helps in the fulfillment of the dance. In her own famous dance "yoga-etude" she has presented a series of sixteen asanas.[3]

Dance is an expression of innate creative power, that is known as Kundalinì. The activity of life force in universe is the cosmic dance which is constantly being done by universal power. Awakening of Kundalini also manifests as a creativity in an artist. In the case of dance, the dancer through the gestures realizes the nectar of Bliss which arises from the union of Siva Sakti, the perfect couple of universe. We close this point with the words of a dancer. "Siva and Parvati have been the inspiration of all dances, the perfect male-female, the dual personalization of the Absolute".[4]

B. Music:

Like dance, music is also a divine manifestation of universal Energy, Kundalinì. The core of music is Nàda, which is one of the aspects of Kundalinì, that is Nàdamayee.

Perfection bestows bliss. In music perfection rests in the Nada tattva. When a singer gets identification with Nàda Sakti, he enjoys the same bliss as a yogi or the dancer feels at the peak of perfection. The Nàda Sàdhanà awakens the latent potentialities of Sàdhaka. How it awakens, that is expressed by Svàmì Prajnananada. "It is the fact when the Sadhaka, artist and the sympathetic listeners realize the real essence of the Nada tattva, they dive deep into the mysterious kamakala or Kundalinì and come to know or urge for knowledge of the ideal of music, stirs the sleeping coiled Kundalini or subconscious mind, and consequently, gives a start for the ascent of the divine basic energy. Gradually the awakened energy penetrates all the force centres of the body (of the spinal cord) and finally reaches the thousand petalled lotus of the Sahasràra, the seat of all consciousness, Parama Siva and then sadhaka artist and the sincere music listeners feel divine communion of the jivatma and the paramàtmà. They then attain the fruition of the Nàda Sàdhanà, which enables them to cut as under the knots of nescience and realize the transcendental Brahman. And this stage can be said to be the ultimate achievement (param prapti) of the practice of music."[5]

This leads us to conclude that liberation through music lies in the realization of the Nàda tattva. The Nàda tattva which is core of music is also an unavoidable aspect of the Tantra system. When we are going to discuss music as the applied side of Tantra, it will not be out of place to have a glimpse of Nàda tattva.

(i) *Theory of Nàda :*

Like Vedic philosophy, Tantra also believes in the world of name and form. (Nàmarupatmàka jagat. As far as the world of name is concerned, Nàda is its essence. Sabda which is the essence of either, is the manifestation of Nàda tattva. Like Ether, being an originator of it, Nàda tattva is also all pervading entity. It is the first modification of ultimate Reality.

There is nothing in this world which has no name. Because very creation depends on name. Volition (Echà) of creation is prior to any concrete creation. Universe was first Willed by Cosmic Creator (Sa asàkàyata) then creation took place. Our willing can be expressed only through words or letters. That's why lord Himself has said in Veda that the creation has come out from speech or vàk. She is the creator of universe.[6] It further declares. "The knower of the Vedas knows that the world is a manifestation of Vàk."[7]

Now let us see how music views Nàda tattva. In the Samgita Darpana, Nàda tattva is highly esteemed, as everthing depends on Nàda. Nàda or Sound is the essence of either which is first among all objects of the world. So it is said that all gross objects are made up of Nàda or sound and hence Nàda is the source of the universe.

The root of the word Nàda, is Nad means the unstruck voice (Anàhata Nàda). This unstruck voice manifests in notes, sentence or language which is known as struck voice (Ahata Nada) because while speaking the outgoing air strikes the vocal chord and creates sound which is classified by Tantric seers as "struck-voice" (Àhata Nàda) These two types of Nadas are also mentioned by the Samgita Darpana and Samgita Makaranda.[8]

For Tantra struck voice (Àhata Nàda) is Vaikhari, one fo the stages of Vàk. The rest stagers are known as Parà, Pasyanti and Madhyama, and unstruck voice (Anàhata Nàda) is a para va. A musician starts his Sàdhanà from struck voice and gradually develops this music to attain the goal, that is unstruck voice, or Anàhata Nàda, or vaikhari to Parà vàk. Now we shall see something about the concept of Nàda according to Tantra.

(ii) *Concept of Nàda in Tantra:*

Awakening of kundalinì is the core of Tantra Sàdhanà. When the Kundalninì awakens, a yogi hears the unstruck voice (Anàhata Nàda). This happens only when prana [vital force] flows from Susumnà instead of Idà and Pingalà. A great radiance arises from Nada which manifests as Bindu or dot. This Bindu is divided into three aspects, that is, namely, will ieeha, knowledge (jñàna) and action (kriyà). Hence, Nàda tattva, the all pervading entity becomes source of will, knowledge and action which are the pre-requirement of every creation.

In Tantra, Bindu is considered as highly potential. As a drop of semen (vìrya) cast into ovum and united with female ova can result into a creation of a new personality or as a seed has a potentialitity to result in a huge tree. likewise, the Nàda which is the same as Bindu is highly potential. Tantra sees no difference between Nàda and Bindu.[9] Svàmì Prajñànanada has quoted a beautiful verse which declares the characteristics and significance of Nàda.[10]

From this we can conclude that the Nada of music is but the reflection of Tàntric notion of Nàda. Nada is the soul of music but for the manifestation of soul, body is required. Soul Nàda manifests through the body Ràga. Ràga is the means through which Nàda manifests. Being a container, Ràga also plays prominent role in music. So let us have a glance over the theory of Ràga.

(iii) *Theory of Ràga:*

Raga is the body of soul Nàda, which means through Ràga, Nàda manifests. What is the meaning of Ràga ? One may have a question. In the treatise on music, Ràga is considered as something that colours the mind with some definite feeling a wave of passion or emotion.[11] Each and every Ràga has potentiality to create some emotions or feelings both in the singer and the listener.

But how Ràga originator. Many theories have been given for this. Some of them lay stress on their base in the Tantric lengendary god, Siva and Sakti, in which they are accepted as the creator of Ràgas. Amongst all Ragas six are considered as major Ràgas.[12] Which are namely, *Sri Raga, Vasanta, Bhairva, Pancama, Megha* and *Natanàràyana.* It is believed that first five ragas are emanated from the Siva Tandava while the last raga came out from the mouth of Pràvàti, Sakti, when She performed the lsya dance. Many difference of opinions are found regarding ascribed to siva or natraja. The origin of the science of music and drama, Siva, the cosmic dancer is known as the arc dramatist and the whole of the Nàtya Sàstra (embracing singing, dancing and dramatic representation) is derived by ancient legend from this great agod (Mahà-deva). According to this legend, the ràgas are said to have been derived from the union of Siva and Sakti (female energy) Pràvati or Giri-jà. From the five faces of Siva at the beginning of His dance (Nrattàrambh) came out of five ragas—Sri ràga, Vasanta, Bhairava, Pancama and Megha. While the sixth ràga Nàt-Nàràyani came out of the sixth mouth of Pàrvatì (Gir-Jàya), the daughter of the Himalaya, when she performed the elegant lasya.[13] Like Samgita Darpana, Suresh Chandra banerjee also accepts the Tantric god siva as the originator of ràgas. In his own words, "Siva and Sakti are the two fundamental principles of the Tàntric philosophy. In the musical lore, too, there is a tradition that Ràgas and Ragains which form the basis of vocal music, emanated respectively from Siva and Sakti. According to one tradition one ràga emanated from each mouth of Siva and one ràga from the mouth of Sakti.[14]

When music is highly related with Tantra, then let us see whether ragas have any relation with centres, (cakras) ascribed by Tantra, or not ? If it is so, how they are related ?

(iv) *Ràgas with reference to centres or cakras:*

The gross universe has come out from the five gross elements (Panca mahà bhùta) namely, earth, water, fire, air and ether. In the world of name (Vànamaya jagat) these elements are represented by the seed letters, lam, Yam, Ram, Vam and Ham respectively. These

Five faces of siva		*Premordial element*	*Bija Mantra*	*Cakra*	Rága
1.	Sadyyojáta	Earth	Lam	Muladhara	Sri Rága
2.	Vamadeva	Water	Vam	Swadhisthana	Vasanta
3.	Aghora	Fire	Ram	Manipura	Bhairava
4.	Tat-Purusa	Air	Yam	Anahata	Pancama
5.	Isana	Ether	Ham	Visuddha	Megha

seed letters are inscribed on the five centres of energy (cakra) in the subtle body which are namely, Mulàdhàra, Swàdhisthàna, Manipura, Anàhata and Visuddha cakra. One of the five gross elements along with the rest is predominant in each of the centres respectively, i.e. earth along with other elements is predominant in Muladhara Water in Swadhisthana etc. Not only centres, elements is predominant in Muldhara Water in Swàhistahàna etc. Not only centres, elements and seed letters but the musical five major ragas are also believed to be related with the five centres of energy. Svami Prajñànànanda has worked out the chart which runs as follows:

Among the five centres, the Visuddha cakra has been considered as the abode of Saraswati. The goddess of music. This centre which is also known as lotus has a sixteen petals from which the sixteen musical notes are produced which are namely : (1) Pranava (the mystic syllable om), (2) Udgitha (a portion of Samveda,' (3) Humphat (Mystic syllable used in incantation, (4) Vausat, (5) Svadha and (6) Svahà (Exclamation used in offering oblation to the deity), (7) namas the term used in connection with the name of diety to signify veneration), (8) Amrita (ambrosia). The seven musical notes namely (9) Shadaja, (10) Rishabha, (11) Gandhara, (12) Madhyama, (13) Pancama, (14) Dhaivat, (15) Nisada, (16) Bisha (poison).*

Rapport with Nàda, (Nàdànusandhàna) is a unique gift given by Tantra for salvation. As we know and feel that mind is very unsteady. In Sàdhanà, mind is required to be fully concentrated and calmed. Tantra says that music is the easiest way through which one can easily concentrate one's mind. This has been beautifully explained in the Nadabindu upanisad.[16]

This lead us to conclude that, the Nàda Sàdhanà of music can be the means of awakening the Kundalini Sakti. Thus music is one of the Tàntric way of realizing the identity between the macrocosm and the microcosm.

C. Astrology:

Suppose that one car is going on with the speed of 120 km. and suddenly the driver, suffers from a hallucination, sees, as if there is dusty board with "Stop, danger ahead" inscribed on it. Driver stops the car and in his great astonishment there is a big valley just a few kilometers from his car. Then he tries to find out the board but in his utter surprise there is no board at all. In this situation what would be think ? This event can be judged differently as depending upon one's mental state and his conception.

It is certain that when he sees a valley near him, he definitely first of all, would think that he is saved miraculously. A theist views this event as a grace of god. A scientist would certainly think that he is saved accidentally while an astrologer sees the impact of planetary system behind this event. But all these views cultimate to one point, that is, there is something which is invisible yet effective. A theist considers it as a grace good or a scientist considers as a mere accident, while for an astrologer it is an influence of planetary system. Tantra considers this 'something' as an influence of energy. How it considers that, we will explain in the sequel. But before we do that let us be aware of the relationship between Tantra and Astrology.

The title given in the beginning of this point declares that astrology is derived from the Tantra. Now let us see which are the common points between these two aspects.

Astrology is based on astronomy. In astrology, it is believed that each and every object feel impact of astron (stars-planet). This is nothing but the reflection of the Tàntric principle of identification between macrocosm and microcosm. Whatever is in universe also exist in human body.

Because of this identification, Tantra considers body as a miniature universe and univore as a body of Siva. The universe which lies in the body can only be seen by the yougic vision. In the cosmic vision (Visvarùpa darsana) Lord krisna has shown to Arjuna the fourteen bhuvanas in Him. Each and every person has got this type of potentialities but its expression requires Sadhana.

Swami Vijanananda in the foreword of the Brhatjatakam very beautifully reflects the base of astrology as resting on vedantic principles which are exactly same as those of Tantra system. Let us see in his own words, "There are two broad and rational priciples on which astrology is based. The first principle upon which the science of Astrology rests, is that of Vedànta, that the whole universe is actually what the term implies a unity; and that a law which is found in manifestation in one portion of the universe must also be equally operative throughout the whole. While the heavens form the macrocosm, man is the microcosm, Each man is a little world exactly representing the universe. While all seem quiet without there is an active world within. Such a world is visible to the inner sight of a yogi. These laws which are operative among the planetary bodies are also in force amongst ourselves.

The second principle is that, by a study of the motion and relative positions of the planets, the operations of these laws may be observed, measured and determined."[17]

Common principles between two systems do not necessarily lead us to conclude that one is derived from another. When we say A is dervied from B, it means A necessarily pre-exists in B. If we apply this fact Tour title, it suggests Tantra is much older than astrology in terms of antiquity. Now let us try to see this.

Veda can be divided into six limbs which are known as Vedànga. They are namely phonetice (Siksà), Rules for sacrificial acts (kalpa), Meter (Chanda), Etymology (Nirukkta), Grammar (Vyakarana) (Vyàkarana) and Astrology (Jyotisa). In the Brahtjàtakam these limbs are equated with the six limbs of Veda purusa in which Jyotisa or astrology is considered as the eyes of Veda purusa.[18]

Veda is the gift of the Àryan people. In the "antiquity of Tantra" with the help of the reports of excavation of Harappà, we have tried to prove that the Tantric germs were deeply rooted into the soil of India before the Àryan came into India. So being a limb of Veda, astrology has a later origin than Tantra. This fact leads us to infer that Àryans might have borrowed the Tàntric principle of identification of microcosm and macrocosm and also of the influence of energy. They might have modified it and applied it in the field of astrology.

How the influence of energy takes place, for this we have to see the theory of atoms and its magnetic currents.

This universe, including physical body and planetary systems have been made out of five elements (Panca Mahàbhùta). Any object can be reduced into atom which is nothing but full of electricity or energy. Sir James Jeans, with the help of researches made by Ruther Ford establishes this tact. "Thanks mainly to the researches of Ruther Ford, it has now been established that every atom is built up entirely of negative charged electrons, and of positive charged particles "Protons"; matter proves to be nothing but a collection of particles charged with electricity.[19]

This atom is nothing but the little magnet. Swami Abhedananda has tried to prove this with aid of the Newton's law and from this, he has also logically derived the fact that being a combination of atoms, human body and earth etc. are also a big magnet.[20]

In previous paragraph while explaining the constitution of universe, we have made reference of five gross elements (Paùca Mahabhuta) among them ether is the most subtle one, and also all pervading entity. From this we can say that in universe, there is nothing like Vacuum but is only an ocean of ether. Planets are very far from human territory. They are not dead but gigantic magnets. Sun is the soul of the planetary system around which the whole system rotates. This system has its own velocity and motion distributing their magnetic currents in the ocean of ether. Being a magnet we also throw the currents in the ocean of either. Harmony between these two currents creates favourable results and disharmony results into misfortune. How this happens is described by Padhey, S.K., in his book "Astrology".[21] All these things establish that being a magnet, planets do have their impact on worldly objects. It is also, at the same time, interesting to note that all planets do not have one and the same type of influence. Some planets are considered as hot, i.e., Mars, Jupiter, Sun while some are as cold namely Moon, Saturn etc. Their impact is felt according to their nature.

Like planets, there is another significant concept in astrology,

COSMIC CONNECTION

Plexus	Letters	Elements (Tridosa)	Planet	Cosmic	Gem	Human system	Nature
1. Múládháara	Vam; Sam: Sam; Sam	Pitta	Mars	Yellow	Coral	Marrow	Hot
2. Swadhisthana	gam; bham; man; yam ram; lam;	Papha with much yáyu	Moon	Orange	Pearl	Blood	Cold
3. Manipura	dam; dham; nam tam; tham; dam; dham; nam; pam; pham	Pitta	Sun	Red	Ruby	Bone	Hot
4. Anáhata	kam; kham; gam; gham; nam; cam; cham; jam; jham;nam; tam; tham	Vata	Saturn	Violet	Blue	Nerves	Cold
5. Visuddha	am; am; eam; im; im; aim; yam; ym; om; rm; oum; lam; rm' m; ham oum;lam; rm; m; ham	Váta &	Venus	Indigo	Diamond	Sperm	Cold
6. Ajna	Ham; ksm	Kapha Sapphire	Jupiter	Blue	Yellow	Fat	Hot
7. Sahasrara	All letters	All the three elements	Mercury	Green	Emerald	Flesh	Cold

This chart is teken from the 'Illustrated Weekly of India, Vol. II, August 29, 1982 by Kadarnath, with title modifivation from original.

that of zodiac, which in terms of Indian astrology known as Ràsi. These are twelve in number and they are considered as the limbs of the body of the kàla purusa or Time-person. The twelve zodiac namely, Mesa, Vrisabha, Mithuna, Karkat, Simha, Kanyà, Tulà, Vriscika, Dhanu, Makara, Kumbha and Mina are related with head, face, chest, heart; belly, waist, pelvis, secrets, two thighs, two knees, two legs, and to feets respectively.

In galaxy, these zodiacs are made out of constellations. There a re twenty-seven in number and each has got four feel. These are equally divided amongst the twelve zodiacs. Each planet rules over one or more zodiacs, i.e. Mars rules over Mesa and Vriscika, Venus rules over Vrisabha and Tulà. Mercury rules over Mithuna and Kanya. Moon rules over Karkat. Sun rules over Simha. Jupiter rules over Dhanu and Mina and Saturn rules over Makara and Kumbha.

Our body also feels the impact of zodiac system on that part which is ascribed in the body of Time-person. For instance, impact of Mesa on head. Vrisabha on face etc. When a malefic planet is in any sign, the part of the body characterised by that sign gets afflicted. And when a benefit planet rules any sign then the corresponding part of the body work effectively.

All these things leads us to believe that the influence of the planetary system on body-mind is an unavoidable aspect of life.

The influence of planets on particular constituents of body (sapta dhatus) and also their connection with three humours of body (Tridosa) can be seen from the given chart. In this chart, relation betwen centres, gros elements, planets etc. have been mentioned which is published in August, 1982 issue of the Illustrtated Weekly of India, which is adopted here with little modification . Here letters, which are ascribed on the centres, are added, which is not given in the original chart, with a view to work out the hypothesis regarding the therapeutic aspect which is referred to in conclusion.

D. Sacrraments :

It was the belief of primitive an that they were surrounded by super natural powers which were their cause of pleasure and pain. In the previous concept, that is of Astrology, we could see that because of the relation of identification between macrocosm and microcosm, we feel the impact of universal forces. And hence, on the important occasions of life, for benign influence of powers, which were termed as deities were and still being invoked.

The Hindus Social System has accepted some occasions of life as important which are sixteen in number which is known as sixteen sacraments (Sodasa Samskàra). Tantra has also accepted the concept of Sacrament but unlike, the former system, it has accepted only ten basic sacraments.

The Mahànirvàna Tantra is the source of the Tàntric concept of sacrament. But one may have a question why sacrament should be performed ? What is the purpose behind it ? The Mahànirvàna Tantra (M.N.T.) views the sacrament as a means of physical-mental purification.[22]

Which are the ten sacraments prescribed by the M.N.T. ? These sacraments are namely (1) conception, (2) pregnancy, (3) simantonnayana, (4) birth, (5) giving the childs name, (6) it's first view of the sun, (7) first eating, (8) tonsure, (9) investiture and (10) Marriage.[23]

What should be done before the celebration of these sacraments ? The M.N.T. has laid down some rules and regulations for it. According to it before performing any sacraments, the kausandika rite is necessary to be performed, in which the lord fire is asked for protection and boons. Lord Brhaspati is also requested for the protection of sacrifice.[24] Lord Indra, Agni, maruta, Brahma, Vasus, Rudras and Prajàpati should be worshipped for grace which may give prosperity.[25] All these things should be performed in prescribed manner for success in the beginning of sacraments.[26] Now we shall see the brief description of all sacraments given by the Mahànirvàna Tantra.

(i) *Garbhàdhàna Samskàra : Conception:*

In this sacrament, the different deities are requested to give good child. First five deities (pañca deva) namely Brahmà, Durgà, Ganesa etc. should be worshipped. After that eight powers (Asta Sakti) should be propitiated. In this sacrament, Lord Visnu is also asked to grant the power to conceive. Tvastrà, for giving the limbs to the child. And Dhàtà is requested to give power to bear.[27] Then Sinivali, Sarasvati and Asvinas are asked to support the womb.[28] And at the end of ceremony, Visnu is again propitiated for excellent son.

(ii) *Pumsavanana Samskarà : Pregnancy :*

This sacrament takes place after the third month of conception. After finishing the daily duties, the husband should worship deities. After this, the wife is asked to drink the special type of curd which is made out of cow's milk. Then the kurca bija Hum and Màyà bija Hrìm is recited for the protection of womb from ghost, pretas and pisàcas[29] (malignant spirit).

(iii) *Simantonnayana Samskàra:*

This rite should be performed in the sixth or eighth month of pregnancy. The same rite takes place as it is mentioned in the putha savnana sacrament. Moreover, three oblations to Visnu, Sùrya and Brahamà should be offered. And then it is requested to Visva-Karma for safe delivery.[30]

(iv) *Jata-karma Samskàra : Birth:*

This rite takes place immediately after the birth of a son. The father performs a Dhàràhoma and gives live oblations to Agni, Indra, Prajàpati, Visvadevas and Bramà for vigour, vitality and firmness of child.[31]

(v) *Nàma-karana Samskàra : Giving the child's name:*

This sacrament should he performed after the sixth or eighth month of birth in the case of son. While in the case of girl, this takes place immediately after Birth. In this sacrament, all rivers are asked to bestow grace for the attainment of Dharama, Artha and Kàma.[32]

Then five oblatios are given to Agni, Vàsava, (Indra), Prajapati, Visva-devas and Brahmà. After that, father takes his son in his lap and speaks his (boy's) name into the right ear.[33]

(vi) *Niskramana Samskàra: Its first view of the sun:*

For a daughter there is no Niskramana Samskàra.[34] But in the case of boy, this should be performed in the fourth or sixth moth after birth.

In this rite, after having attended daily duties, the father should, after bathing worship Ganesa and then son should be bathed adorned with clothes and jewels. Then his father requests Brahamà, Visnu, Siva, Durgà, Indra, Vàyu, Agni, Varuna for the protection whenever he goes out from the house. Then, father takes his child to show the sun.[35]

(vii) *Anna-pràsanna Samskàra: First eating*

When the child becomes six or eight months old, this, rite should be done. First of all dieties are worshipped. Then father should meditate on the devi Annadà (Giver of food) and offer her five oblations. After that pàyasa (Rice boiled in milk with sugar and a little ghee) should be put into the child's mouth by uttering the Mantra of oblation of five vital airs.[36] Then a little rice and curry should be put in the child's mouth.

(viii) *Cùdàkarma Samskàra : Tonsure :*

This sacrament takes place at the age of third or fifth year. All deities should be worshipped first. Then after performing all rites given in the scriptures, the father should request to omnipresent creator for well-being of a child.[37]

(ix) *Upanayana Samskàra : Investiture:*

This sacrament takes place at the age of eight. After perfroming the rite given in the scriptures, the guru gives him a knotted girdle. Then boy should pronounce, "'Hirim', may this auspicious girdle be propitious".[38] Then the sacrificial thread is given to child. After this, the oblations are offered to all dieties. Then guru whispers the pranava mantra (Aum) in the right ear of a child. Guru, then, recites The Gàyatri Mantra for the attainment of progress of a child in life.[39]

(x) *Udvàha Samskàra*: *Marriage*:

In this sacrament, first of all, all deities are worshiped. Then after having completed all rites in the scripture, Lord Prajapati is asked for the accomplishment for the desires of newly wedded couple. Then at the end of the ceremony, devi Raja-Rajesvari, Kali, Bhuvanesvari etc. are requested for the protection of couple.[40]

Thus, the decrition here given shows that on every occasions of life, deities are invoked for the benign influence and also for the removal of evil impacts. Here we have mentioned only that part of the sacrament which is directly related with the influence of energy. And rest of the part which is related with ritual is omitted.

2. Conclusion:

The contents of this chapter point out the widespread area of life which is influenced by the Tàntric principles. Man is not merely an animal but he is something more than that. That something is expressed by his cultural, religious, social activities like arts, sacraments etc. Tantra has not left this area also. Its principles, namely influence of energy, identification between macrocosm-microcosm, the concept of mind-body purification etc. are largely applied in all these activities. How these principles are applied in dance, music, astrology and sacraments that we have already seen in this chapter.

All these above mentioned aspects are also can be utilized as health giving techniques. In the definition of healthy body-mind complex, many factors are to be considered. Among then flexibility of body and calmnes of mind are the deciding ones. Dance gives both of these. In dance, dancer has to do various types of backward, forward, sideward movements which keeps body flexible. Secondly, dance gives health like the Hathayogic postures (Àsanàsa). The dancing mudràs have great resemblance with postures. So while, doing mudràs, a dancer does àsanàsa automatically, which give him/her therapeutic results. So dance makes body free from diseases by keeping it in constant movements.

Not only movement of body but in dance, expression (Bhava) also is very significant. If suppose a dancer is presenting an expression of Ràdha, he/she becomes one with Ràdha. This identification with only one concept cultivates the power of concentration which prevents the wastage of mental energy which generally flows through the various modifications of mind. It help keeping one away from distortion of mental energy and thus keeps one mentally healthy.

Like dance, music also secures the therapeutic value. Music gives calmness to mind to both singer and listener. This calmnes of mind is highly required when most of our diseases arise out of mental tension.

As being a resemblance with the Hathayogic postures, dancer gets its therapeutic result. Likewise, a musician gets the healing effects of prànàyàma. The therapeutic value of prànàyàma needs no example. As we know prana and mind go together. By controlling one, other can automatically be controlled. So if the speed of pràna is under control, becomes steady and concentrated.

In the presentation of Ràga, the practice of Kumbhaka, (retention of air) is highly beneficial. So for being a good singer, it is prerequirement to have control over technique of Prànàyàma. This practice of Pranayama prevents the ailments of Nàdis-bodily channels which makes body undiseased and healthy. The Ghernada Samhita also supports this view by declaring that, the regular practice of Kumbhaka keeps body-mind healthy.

The role of astrology in are of therapeutic is different than that of dance and music. It not only gives the aapy Therapybut it also predicts the diagnosis of diseases. How it does so ?

In the chart attached in the concept of astrology we saw the connection between letters, Tàntric centers, human system, Tridosa element etc. From all these connection we can construct one hypothesis which runs as follows:

As we know the place of zodiac in the Indian astrology is very significant. Different letters are ascribed to all zodiacs. If suppose subject A is born under the influence of Aries. The letters ascribed to Aries are A.L.I. According to the chart, A is related with Visuddha cakra, L is with Swàdhisthàna cakra while E again with Visuddha cakra. If we apply the Tridosa elements which are related with this cakras, we can say that, this subject may have a constitution of Vàta and Kapha. He may be subject to that diseases which are related with the constitution of Vàta and Kapha. This hypothesis can be applied in the area of all zodiacs.

Secondly, it also gives the prediction of diseases by considering the movement of planetary system. Every being born under one sign or zodiac which is governed by one planet. There are nine planets, in system which are inter-related either with the relation of friend, enemy or neutral. In the movement of planets, if suppose a planet comes in a sign which has a relation of enemy with the Lord of the zodiac, it gives unfavourable results to the subject. So from the calculation of the movement of planets it can be predicted the favourable or unfavourable time of a subject for the treatment of the disease to which one is subject. To prevent the evil influence which are arise from the disharmony certain Mantras are prescribed. Removal of evil influence also can be done by wearing pearl, gem, diamond etc., but should be properly charged with Mantras otherwise, it would not give any results. So thus astrology and therapy are linked with Tàntric practices with a view to diagnze correctly the diseases and to prescribe proper remedy for disease.

Like dance, music and astrology, sacraments also secure healing value. As the Mahànirvfàna Tantra declares, sacraments are designed for the purification of mind-body. That purified body-mind complex is the source of health.

As we have see all sacraments should be done with the help of Mantras and sacrifice (yajña), Pollution of atmosphere, which is also one of the cause of diseases, can be removed by the vibration of Mantras and flame of fire of sacrifice (yajña). This pollution less atmosphere gives health to subject and the people living around it.

This is how Tantra is mainly preoccupied not only with spiritual uplift of the individual but also his physical well being. The basic assumption of Tantra is not only yoga or mediation but bhoga or enjoyment also. Only yoga leads one to abstraction and away from life while only bhoga or indulgence in worldly affairs weakens the body-mind. Tantra by uniting yoga and bhoga makes life purposeful and worth living.

FOOTNOTE

1. Rao, Gopinath T.A., Elements of Hindu Iconography, Vol. II, Part I, p. 23, The Law Printing House, Madras, 1916.

2. Woodroffe, John, Quoted by Banerji Projensh, Dance of Shiva, p. 30, First Edition, 1942, Kitabistan, Allahabad.

3. "Yoga" Jounal, April, 1978, Vol. XVI, No. 4, Published by Bihar School of Yoga , Monghyr.

4. Sàràbhai Mrinalini, Understanding the Bharat Natyam, p. 29, Maharaja Sayaji Rao University, 1965.

5. Svàmì Prajnanananda, A historical study of Indian Music, Preface-XXVIII.

6. Vàgeva Visvà bhuvanani jajñe vaca iti I

Sa Sarvamamrutam yaea martyamiti srutihi

Thakur, Omkarnath, Pranava Bharti (Hindi),p. 4, N. M. Tripathi and Company, First Edition 1956.

7. Sabdasya parinamosyamitiàmnày vido vidugh I

Ibid, p. 4.

8. Nàdena Vyajyate Varnah padam varnàt padàdvacah I

Vacaso Vyavahàrosyam nàdàdhinamidam jagat

Samgit Darpana 1/14, Taken from Pranava Bharti by Tahakur Omkarnath, p. 1.

9. Yo vai nada so vai binduh I

yogini hridayam.

Chattopadhaya, Kshetresachandra, Published by Director, Research institute, Varanasi, Second Edition, 1963.

10. Svàmì Prajñànananda, A historical study of Indian Music, p. 312, First Edition, 1975.

11. —Ranjayati iti Ragà I

Definition and translation taken from "Ràgas and Ragnis" by Ganguli, O.C., p. 1, Nalanda Publication, 1935.

12. Ràgà: Sadayah I

Pancamasara Samhita—Nàrada.

13. Siva sakti samàyogat ràgànà sambhvobavet

Pancasyat Pancaràgàhà myu: Sasthantu Girijàmukhàt I

Madyovkràntu Sriràgo vamadevàd Vasantakah I

Aghorat bhairavad bhùtatpurusat Pancamosbhavat

Isànàkhyonmeghràgo nàtyàrambhe Sivàdbhùta I

Girijaya mukhat flasyae natanarayano bhvat I

Samgita Darpana, Translation and verse taken from 'Raga and Ragini' by Ganguli, O.C., pp. 23-24.

14. Banerjee S. C, Fundamentals of ancient Music and Dance; p. 78, L.D. Series 57, First edition, 1976.

15. Tagore, S.M., Universal history of music, Appendix, p. IV, The Chowkhamba Sanskrit Studies, Vol. XXXI, Published by the Chaukhamba Sanskrit Series Office, Varanasi, Second Edition, 1963.

16. Yatra Kutrapi và nàde...

Citam Viliyate I

Nàdabindupanisad 38 to 44.

17. Swami, Vijñànanda, The Brihàtjataka of Varàha Mihira, p. 1, Foreword, Oriental Books Reprint Corporation, Delhi 1979. Second Edition.

18. Sabdasàstram mukham jyotisam caksusì

Srotramuktam niruktam can kalpa karou I

Yatu Sikshàsya vedasya sà nàsika pàdapada-

dvyam cada àdaihbudhaih II Ibid, p. 2.

19. Jeans, James, The mysterious universe, p. 46, Cambridge University Press, 1945.

20. Swami, Abhedananda, Complete works of Swami Abhedanauda, Vol. VI, p. 67, Ramkrishna Vedanta Matha, 1968.

21. Padhey, S. K., Astrology, pp. 7 to 10.

22. Samskàrena vinà devi deha sudhihrna jàyate I

Nà samskrutoadhikàrì syàd daive pitre ca karmani

M.N.T. Chapter 2, Edited by Avalon Arthur, Vol. XIII, Motilal Banarisdass, 1977.

23. Jìvasekah pumsavana sìmantonnyanam tathà I

Jàtanàmnì niskra mannnàsanmatah param I

Cudupanayanaodvàhàh samskàràhà kathità dasa II

The Mahànirvàna Tantra 9-4.

24. M.N.T. 9-33.

25. M.N.T. 9-68.

CHAPTER - 5

HUMAN ANATOMY AND TANTRA

CHAPTER - 5

1. Introduction:

Physical body is the main gate for approaching the soul. In the body, Lord who controls the entire universe also is present. Lord in a form of power lies dormant in body. In a course of time, through constant efforts and though yogic practices, man unfolds his latent powers. The physical body is the reservoir of energy and the only means for the unfoldment of which is the goal of the sàdhaka. And because of this, body is not given for the unholy purpose or only for the enjoyment of sensual pleasrues. The prime purpose is to attain liberation from limitations of body and mind, and attainment of spirituality through body.

Physical frame, in the Tantra system, is highly esteemed as the temple of Spirit or God (Dehao devalayo devi). And hence, it should be kept pure and perfect in condition. The process of Tantra sàdhanà starts from gros and ends into subtle. And hence it has accpted physical body positively. Miercea Eliade with the reference of the Gheranda Samhita declares that, "The body is no longer the source of pain, but the most reliable and effective instrument at man's disposal for `conquering death'. And since liberation can be gained even in this life, the body must be preserved as long as possible and in perfect condition, precisely as an aid on meditation."[1]

The Rasàrnavam, the another Tàntric treatise also supports the positivitly of the body. As it views, it is of no use if liberation is gained after death. Even donkey can also get it. So in order to attain liberation in this life, the preservation of body is very essential.[2]

For Tantra, the preservation of body can be prolonged according to the will power or desire through the Hathayogic àsanàsa, pranàyàma, Tàntric techniques and also by the intakes of mercury preparations.

Physical diseases and mental ailments are hurdles in the way of longetivity. There are various ways and means through which one can overcome these hurdles. They are known as various therapies. Healthy body-mind complex is the goal of all therapies. Any therapy, is first applied on the physical body and it ultimately affects the mind. So different therapies have worked out the anatomy. At present Allopathy, Àyurveda, Homeopathy etc., are the leading ones. Tantra also has beinf a thereapy its own view regarding anatomy. It is really a very surprising to note that the anatomy which is worked out, in the twentieth century with the help of the scientific instruments, largely tallies with the Tantra anatomy which is revealed out in hoary past.

In this chapter an attempt has been made to present the anatomy given by Tantra and Allopathy. The concluding portion covers the synthesis of the both. We shall, first, briefly survey the anatomy of Allopathy.

A. *Anatomy given by the Allopathy System:*

The literature of the anatomy given by the Allopathy system is very large, hence, it is difficult to present it here in detail. This system has accepted nine main system for the sustenance of body which are namely. (1) Bones, (2) Muscles, (3) Digestion, (4) Circulation, (5) Respiration, (6) Excretion, (7) Nervous, (8) Glands and (9) Reproduction.

All these system have significant place in the maintenance of the body but here we shall mention only the nervous system and the gland system as they are directly related with the Tantra anatomy.

(i) *The Nervous System:*

The nervous system is connected with all bodily systems because it controls all activities which are going on in the body.

The nervous system consists of two divisions. (1) Central system and (2) Autonomus system The central nervous system mainly consists of the brain, twelve pairs of cardinal nerves, spinal cord ad forty-three pairs of the spinal nerves. The autonomous nerveous system consists of spinal cord, sympathetic nervous system and the para-sympathetic nervous system.

The spinal cord which is elongated in the shape, is a prolongation of brain, and, is located in the hollow of the spinal column. Spinal nerves start from the spinal cord and issue out from the spinal column. All these forty-three pairs of nerves spread out themselves throughout the body and form a closely woven network.

Functionally, nerves may be divided into two groups. Motor and Sensory or efferent ad afferent respectively. All mascular activities are responsible for motor nerves while the feeling of smell, taste, touch etc., are responsible for sensory nerves.

The autonomous nervous system consists of two rows of ganglian that is group of nerve cells. These two rows of nerves are mutually connected and cross each other at certain points along the spinal cord. These cords on each side of the spinal column are known as sympathetic nervous system and the para sympathetic nervous system.

Life process which is going on in our body, without the interference of our will, is under the control of these systems. They work independently, hence, they are known as autonomous system. The effort of Hathayogi and Tàntric sàdhaka is to make this autonomous system under his will and that way he controls the bodily activities.

(ii) *Gland System:*

In body there are certain organs which themselves secret fluid with their special properties, which help in the action and growth of the body, known as glands. The secretion of glands is known as hormon on which physical-mental growth depends. Long before the Allopathy system has found out the glands, the Hathayoga has advocated exercises for the proper secretion which ultimately result into the growth of body-mind complex.

These glands are known as the ductless glands because they pas their secretions directly into blood and lymph etc. These glands are namely, Pituitary, Pineal, Thyroid, thymus, Pancreas, Adrena and Testes or in case of woman Ovaries.

The ductless glands are situated at the different parts of the body. The Pineal and the Pituitary are situated in the brain. The Thyroid is located in the neck. The Thymus is situated between the neck and the chest. The Adrenals are situated above the kidneys. The Ovaries in the case of female are situated in the pelvic region where as the Testes, the corresponding male reproductive gland are located in the Scrotum.

It has been scientifically found out that the ductless gland secretion very powerfully affects the physiological balance of the body. Hence proper secretion of it enhance the growth of body-mind. Hence proper secretion of it enhances the growth of body-mind and over secretion and under secretion results into abnormalities.

Now after having seen about the Allapathy anatomy, let us turn our attention towards the Tantra anatomy.

B. *Tantra Anatomy:*

The Tantra anatomy runs round the concept of centres (cakras) and subtle channels (nàdis).

(i) *Theory of six centres:*

The lexical meaning of the term cakra is wheel. Here it denotes the centres of consciousness.[3] Cakras are believed to be situated in the subtle body or pranamaya Sarira where energy is concentrated at the highest level. These centres have a great resemblance with the glands which are located in the physical body. In the gland system, we could see that the secretion of gland affects the growth of body-mind complex. The energy which is required for the growth of body-mind is provided by the centres or cakras. So the concentration on centres automatically effects on the secretion of glands and it ultimately results into healthy body.

Diseases arise when a person is not in a position to distribute the energy properly though centres. Poor digestion, which is considered as the root of all diseases may mean inadequate supply of energy in the navel region or the Manipura cakra.

How many centres are present in the body is still a matter of controversy. An exact figure is still not known to us. All Hathayogic and Tàntric treatise give different numbers. According to some it is nine, for others it is eleven but seven is generally accpted figure and here we also follow that figure. These seven cakras are namely, Mùlàdhàra, Swàdhisthàna, Manipura, Anàhata, Visuddha, Àjñà and Sahasràra cakra.

These centres are also known as lotuses. They contain specific number of petals namely, 4, 6, 10, 12, 16 and 1000 respectively. On every petal Samskrit letter is ascribed. It means, the Mùàadhàra cakra contains four petals hence four letters. The Swàdhistahàna cakra contains six petals hence six letters and so on. The specific number of petals also represents the position of yoga nàids situated around that centre. Now let us see the details of all cakras.

(ii) *Mùlàdhàra cakra:*

In the term 'Mùlàdhàra', 'mùla' means root while 'dhara' means support. It is root of all yogic subtle nàdis and also the supporter of the root of energy, that is, Kundalinì.

This centre is located between the genital and the anus region.[4] This centre contains four petals on which four letters from Vam to Sam are ascribed.

The bìja mantra lam of Prithvi or earth element is predominant here. This is also represented by the elephant or Airàvat. Symbolically as it is the centre of gross physical powers. Elephant is the most powerful among animals and hence it is symbolized by elephant. In this centre, Kundalinì rests on the Svayambhu linga or the root of the genital organ, which is covered by the triangle with down-ward apex, which again is a geomerical representation of gross energy. The triangle is a symbol of all a human powers like power of knowledge, will and action.

(iii) *Swàdhisthana cakra:*

The term 'Swàdhistàhàna' is a combination of two words, that is Swa and adhisthana. Swa means prana while adhisthana means resting place.[5] Hence Swadhisthana means the resting place of prana. This centre is situated at the root of the genital organ.[6] The bija mantra Vam of the water element is predominant here. This six petalled lotus contains the letter from Bam to Lam. The vehicle of this centre is Maker or crocodile. The aspirant who meditates on this centre becomes free immediately, from all his enemies.

(iv) *Manipura cakra:*

This centre is located above the Swàdhisthàna cakra and anatomically at the root of the navel region.[7] The bìja mantra Ram of the fire element is predominant here. It has ten petals on which the letters from Dam to Pham are located. Meditation on this centre makes one free from the fear of fire. Even if he throws himself into fire, he remains alive.

(v) *Anàhata cakra:*

This centre is believed to be situated in the region of heart. The seed letter yam of the element air is predominant here. The vehicle of this centre is antelope. The nature of both antelope and the air is the same, i.e. the fleeting nature. A sadhaka who mediates on this centre controls vayu and is full of capacity either to create or to destroy the world.[*] This claim though seems to be exaggerated, it shows to what an extent the meditator can develop himself. The simily given shows to what an extent the meditator can develop himself. The simily given shows that he virtually becomes as powerful as Lord himself.

(vi) *Visuddha cakra:*

This centre is located in the region of throat. All sixteen vowels are located on this sixteen petalled lotus. Visuddha means pure. Concentration on this centre makes the mind of a sàdhaka pure from all impurities. The bìja mantra Ham of the ether element is predominant here. Meditation on this centre gives the knowledge of three worlds. It also makes free from diseases and sorrows.[9]

(vii) *Àjñà cakra:*

This centre is located in the body at the space between the

two eyebrows. The bija mantra Aum is located here. This centre is a seat of mind. The mind of a sadhaka receives the commands (Àjñà) of guru through the concentration on this centre. Concentration on it also destroys the past deeds of sadhaka and he becomes jìvanamukta. It is equated as a third eye of Siva which destroys ignorance as well as desires.

(vii) *Sahasràra cakra:*

The Sahasràra cakra is located at the top of the head. This centre contains sand and petals (Sahasra means thousand). It is the place where the union of Siva-Sakti takes place. Here we should note that, this centre is very subtle in nature and because of this, it is not considered as belong to the plan of body. Because of its subtlety, it is not counted in the six centres.

(viii) *Nàdi: Theory of Channels:*

In Tantra, nàdi does not mean gross channels but it contains subtle energy or prana. These channels are spread throughout the body and hence they are many in number. Because of this, they cannot be counted. Though, however, some figures have been proposed. According to some treatise the figure is 3,00,000 for others, it is 2,00,000. But the figure 72,000 is largely accepted.

Among all these nàdis, ten are important namely, Idà, Pingalà, Susumnà, Gandhàri, Hastajihvà, Pusà, Yasasvini, Àlambusa, Kuhù and Samkhini. The first three, among these are more significant.

Ida and Pingalà are located at the end of the spine. They extend from the end of spine to nostrils. They are considered as the container of the lunar and solar or mental and the vital currents in the body respectively. The Susumnà nàdi is said to be generally closed at the base of the spine and can be opened by certain yogic practices.

Pràna or life force flows either through Idà or through Pingalà generally. The Tantra sàdhaka arrests this way of flowing of pràna and he tries for drawing prana through the Susumnà nàdi.

2. Conclusion:

All therapies revolve round the concept of the physical body. According to Tantra, all organs of the body are connected with cakras or centres through subtle channels or nàdis. The power which is required by the limbs of body is provided by the centres of consciousness throgh nàdis. This concept has a great resemblance with the All pathic concept of glands and the nergous system. We have seen in the anatomy of Allopathy that the growth of body and efficiency of nervous system depends upon proper or balanced secretion of glands.

According to the Tantra, the Mùlàdhàra cakra is situated at the base of the spine of which prithvi or earth element is predominant, the supporter of all things. The Àyurveda sùtràni also declares. the Mùlàdhàra cakra is a supporter of all bodily substance, sapta dhàtus.[10]

To show the predominance of gros element, Tantra declares this centre as the seat of prithvi tattva or earth element. Physiologically, this centre situated at the anus region and is also associated with the area of excretion of solid matter from body.

The Swàdhisthàna cakra is located at the root of the genital organ of which water element is predominant. In body, all output of fluids, i.e. urination and discharges of semen takes place here.

The Manipura cakra is believed to be situated at the navel region which is associated with the fire element. Physiologically when the inner flame of fire (Jatharàgni) is properly regulated, it results into health. Otherwise it can be the source of diseases.

The Anàhata cakra is located at the heart region. This is the centre where the air element is predominant. It is a centre of nutrition. Heart distributes purified blood sent to it by lungs to various parts of the body. The efficiency of lungs is very much needed for the purification of blood. This efficiency of lungs can be increased by prànàyama which is highly related with the air element.

The Visuddha cakra is located in the area of throat. The element ether is predominant here. All vowels are located on this center. Physiologically this centre is considered as the centre of vocalization.

The Àjñà cakra is located between the two eyebrows. It is also known as the third eye. It is the palace of the Pineal gland. This centre controls our desires as well as gives us knowledge. The Pineal gland does this same work according to Allopathy.

The Sahasràra cakra is located at the top of the skull, where the consciousness is evolved at the highest degrees. Physiologically, it is a place of the *Pituitary* gland.

According to the Allopathy, the Pituitary gland is located in between two brains and is known as master gland. Because it controls the function of all other glands. The secretion which it released are important from the point of view of maintenance and destruction of the body. It is a seat of the desire of reproduction also. Hence Tantra has aptly described it as kameswara.

The Tàntric centres and nàdis are very subtle in nature. So it is not proper to identity then with the gross physical system. Here we have mentioned it just to show the resemblance between the two system namely Allopathy and Tantra.

The anatomy which is mentioned by Tantra is very subtle in nature and can be seen only through the yogic vision, and not by the dissection of the body.

FOOT NOTE

1. Eliade, Mircea: yoga—Immortality and freedom. Translated from the French by Willard R. Trask, p. 227, Pollingen sereis LVI, Second Edition, 1969.

2. Pindapàte cayomoksah so ca moksa nirarthakah I
Pinde tu patite devi II gadarbhopi vimucyate
Rasàrnava Tantra 1-9.

3. Cakram saktisamùh I Yoginì hrdaya Cakrasamketa nirupanam, Verse 7, Commentary of Bhàskaracharya on Yoginì hrdaya.

Edited by Chattopadhyaya, Kshetresachandra, Saraswati Bhavan Granthamala, Vol. 7, Second Edition, 1963.

4. Atha àdhàrapadman susumnàsya lagnam dhvajàdho gudrodhva catuh sona patram.
Sat cakranirupanam 4.

5. Sva sabdena bhavet prànah swàdhisthànam tadàsrayam I
Yogacudamani upanisad II

6. Sousumnya madhya ghatitama dhvajamùla dese
Sat cakranirupanam, 14.

7. Tasyord have nàbhimùle dasadala lasite pùrnamegha pràkae.
Sat cakranirupanam.

8. Vàcàmìsvara esvaraspi jagatàm raksà vinàse ksmah I
Sat cakranirupanam, 26.

9. Trikàlànàm darsi sakalahitakase rogasoka pramukta.
Sat cakranirupanam, 31.

10. Nanu yogànispi mùlàdhàra màdibhùtam sakala dhatu posakam petal 3-90.

The Àyurveda Sùtram with commentary of Yognandanàth. Edited by Dr. R. Sharma Sastry, p. 141, Mysore, 1922.

CHAPTER - 6

Healing Aspect of Yantra and Mantra

CHAPTER - 6

1. Introduction:

On this earth among all existing species, human race is the only one which has become victim of the self created disease. Many therapies have been worked out to come over this calamity but still, we are not in a position to remove all diseases. On the contrary, sometimes, the side effects, of drugs appear in a form of new diseases.

The basic reason of the frequent appearance of disease lies in our artificial or unnatural way of living. We do everything to go against nature, e.g. our habit of eating. We must eat whenever we feel the need for it or hunger for it and eat only those thing which we know are conducive to good health. Instead we either eat more out of fashion or eat those things which we know are not conducive to health. This improper way of eating, creates complexities in stomach which result into various diseases. Not only in eating, in our routine life we do many more things which we know, may result into some sort of irregularities either physical or mental.

Besides this, there is also one vital reason which is responsible to create physical-mental and also spiritual disorders, that is, the neglect of the inner healing power or the power of resistance of body against diseases give by nature. Modern life is full of stresses and strains. We are always in hurry and hence we are constantly in search of instant cure and due to this we take such drugs which they cure the disease instantly but ultimately harm the body.

There are many side effects of such drugs, like insomnia, blood pressure, disturbance of sugar balance etc. And therefore, the experts in this field are in search of those drugs which are harmless or in search of drugless therapy.

Yantra and Mantra are techniques designed for cultivating inner latent power of resistance of body-mind with which we are not aware of out of ignorance. We, therefore, wonder when experts in this field talk in terms of superhuman powers. Superior power invoke wonders because we are ignorant of them.

Yantra and Mantra techniques worked out for cultivating latent power of body-mind which are based upon highly ascertainable psychological and spiritual facts. Yantras are formed out of certain geometrical figures like dot, triangle etc. They serve as means of concentration. It is recognized by Tàntrics that concentration of mind is multiplication of mental faculty and addition of mental powers while dissipation of Paycho-physical energy is waste of energy and consequently an invitation to diseases. This process of concentration if perfected, may lead to not only drugless therapy but also increases longevity.

Tàntric of ages have perfected the techniques for concentration. Mantra is again a very powerful weapon in the armoury of Tantra for bringing about highest form of concentration by which the expert simply by concentration of his cultivated powers, can bring about wonderful results with the help of repetition of certain syallbles knwon as seed letters or Bija Mantra. Now let us see the details of Yantra and Mantra with the reference of their therapeutic value.

A. *Yantra Therapy*:

(i) *Introduction*:

One of the theories regarding the creation of world is that, world s nothing but the mere projection of mind . Mind perceives world objects with the help of the data given by the sense organs. So the expansion of vision of mind depends upon the amount of data given by sense organs. For instance, if the sense of hearing, is cultivated more, then the owner of it, can hear more loudly, than another man. Same is the case with all sense. A yogi or a sàdhaka, who has expanded the inner latent ability of sense organs can open the subtle apparatus for the knowledge of the world which is not possible in case of a layman.

Tantra shows us the way of the process of expansion, of the power of senses. One of the meaning of Tantra is expansion (Ötan

= to expand). Tantric techniques are designed for this purpose. If , suppose the powers are aroused by the application of Tantra techniques then what's the use of it, if they are not channelized. Uncontrolled power harms the sàdhaka himself. Considering this, Tantra has devised the unique method of Yantra, The term 'Yantra' comes forms the root 'yam' which means to control. Yantra is an aid for controlling the power.

Yantra is also representation of the Higher Reality. It represents the Reality in a geometrical forms like dot line, triangle etc. These are not merely geometrical sings. They are also Yantric symbols which represent subtle meanings of the Higher Reality.

Sri Yantra, among all the Yantras, is the most auspicious Yantra represents devi or sakti. The formation of the Sri Yantra is unique. Five triangles with downward apex are superimposed by four triangles with downward base. This combination results into forty-three triangles. The outer appearance of these triangles can be classed into seven circles which are considered as the centres of consciousness.

Tantra techniques are based upon sound principles. (1) Unity of microcosm and macrocosm and (2) Identity of two in an individual. Yantra is a means through which this identity can be realized by the individual. Sri Yantra is a symbolic representation of these two principles and hence it represents the human-body-mind complex with self or consciousness as the presiding deity and therefore it functions as a link between these two. It is used as a means for contemplation. Contemplation on it, results into the identification of microcosm and macrocosm. Moreover, concentration on Sri Yantra also gives beneficial rewards to sadhaka.

One of the cakras of Sri Yantra, is Sarvarogahara cakra, remover of all diseases. The concentration on this centre insures the sàdhaka freedom from all diseases. We, therefore, say that Sri Yantra technique has tremendous therapeutic value in insuring himself from all diseases. Like Sri Yantra, there are also other Yantras which are believed to be the means for curing and protecting the sàdhaka from the attacks of physical and mental diseases. In this chapter we shall make reference to two Tàntric treatises namely, the Saundrya Laharì and the Kalpacintamanih for supporting the view.

For the convenience of presenting the details, this chapter has been divided into two groups, A and B. A consists of the details regarding Yantra and its symbolic representation while B contains its therapeutic value. Now let us be acqainted with the meaning and significance of Yantra the first.

(ii) *Yantra and its symbolic meaning:*

In scriptures, which deal with the sàdhanà aspect, the Ultimate Reality is termed as deity (Div=shine) because it is viewed as light. In Tantra, this great effulgence of light is considered as Lord Siva.[1]

According to the science, which deals with the analysis of the rays of the sun, the objects of world are nothing but the various combinations of the rays of light. These rays are seven in number. So by making change into the combinations of rays, any object can be transformed into any other object. Swami Yogananda has mentioned this type of illustration in his, 'autobiography of a yogi' in which his guru had transformed camphor into graphite.

Sun light as the great radiance is formless. When it manifests, it takes form. Yantra represents the Higher Reality and hence whatever is manifested by the Higher Reality, the worldly objects, are Yantras. This view is also expressed by Devaràja Vidya Vàcaspati. As he declares, "there are, in the world, innumerable Yantras. Every shape, every leaf, every flower is a Yantra, which through its shape, its colour, its perfume tells us the story of creation."[2]

Yantra represents Light or the Higher Reality in the form of geometrical figures. Due to this presentation of light, Yantra is considered as the abiding place of deity.[3] The Higher Reality is figured out in symbols or forms because a layman is not in a position to grasp the formless great radiance, so at initial level, to have a glimpse of the Higher Reality, Yantra is required. As the Yoginì Tantra declares , "The goddess is to be worshipped in the sex emblem, a book , a symbolic drawing on the ground, an image, water or a stone."

This leads us to confer that Yantra is a store house of energy or a symbolic representation of the cosmic energy underlying all objects of the universe. Moreover, it is, as Zimmer views, is also an instrument. He gives this view by breaking the term 'Yantra'. The term 'Yantra' is a combination of Yam+tra. Yam means to control while tra indicates instrument. In his own words, "Yantra is an instrument designed to curb the psychic forces by concentrating them on a pattern, and in such a way that this pattern becomes reproduced by the worshipper's visualizing power. It is a machine to stimulate inner visualization, meditation and experiences.[5]

Yantra is formed out by the figures like dot, circle, line, triangle etc. They also contain the subtle meaning underlying the Higher Reality. Now let us proceed with the Symbolic meaning of the various figures.

(iii) ***Symbolic meaning of Yantra:***

In the Veda, there is a beautiful story regarding the omnipresence of Lord. As it says, having created universe, God stood out of the universe and thought about how to penetrate or enter into the universe. Then he decided to enter into the universe through name and form. So wherever there is a name and form (Nàma-Rùpa), the Higher Reality pervades in it.[6] In Yantra, these forms of the Higher Reality are reflected in such a manner that. Throgh contemplation on them, sadhaka can feel the presence of the Higher Reality.

Both the constituents of the Higher Reality, the macrocosm and the microcosm, are the same and they are represented by five gross elements (Pañca mahàbhùta). In Yantra, these forces are symbolized in a figurative manner. So by concentration on it, one can establish harmony between the microcosm and macrocosm.

The geometrical figures, from which Yantra is composed are dot. triangle, circle, square etc. Now we shall see the subtle meanings of them.

a. Dot: Bindu:

Bindu is represented by dot. As the whole of Geometry is an expansion of dot, so also the entire Yantra is an expansion of Bindu. Yantras or geometrical figures are drawn on soil or on Bhùrjapatra or the bark of trees meant for them or on leaves or on copper, silver or gold plates. Various movements going on in cosmos are the creation of various forces working in the cosmos. These forces or movements are symbolically represented on the Yantra.

The cosmic forces are all pervasive and hence represented on Yantra are believed to be all pervasive, e.g. Ether which is all pervasive is represented in the form of Bindu. In Tantra, this dot or Bindu is considered as Siva which symbolically represents the source of creation.

Not only Tàntric seers, but the western psychologist like Jung has also contemplated on this aspect. He has utilized the word 'Mandala' for cakra and coined the word centre of Mandala as Siva In his own word creating in emanation. Siva according to the Tàntric tradition is one existence, the Timeless in its perfect state. Creation begins when this unextended point known as Siva Bindu appears in the eternal embrace of its feminine side, the Sakti."[7]

The expansion of Bindu takes the form of triangle, trikona which according to the Yantra symbolism represents Sakti. Bindu is Siva and trikona is Sakti. In Tantra, both these are considered as identical.[8]

b. Triangle : Trikona :

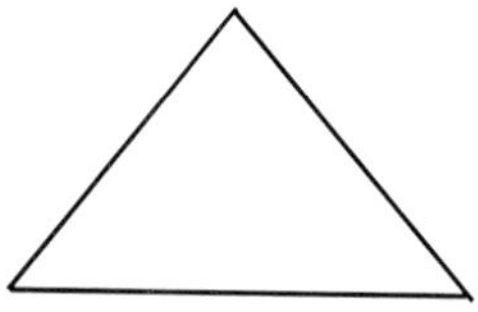

Triangle is an embelm of Sakti and Sakti is, according to the Sanskrit lexicon, considered as of a feminine gender, hence it is also known as yoni or the female reproductive Rogan because the whole cosmos has come out of it. The Rgveda also refers the origin of cosmos as yoni.* There are two types of triangles figured out in Yantra.

One is with upward base while the other is of downward base.

The triangle with apex upward shows the way of sublimation.

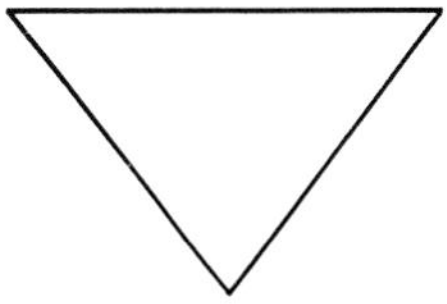

Among the five elements, it represents the fiery element or Agnitattva. As fire goes upward, the aspiration of sàdhaka also goes upward. This triangle is also known as Siva kona.

C. Sakti kona.

The triangle with apex downward represents the water element or Àpa tattva. The tendency of water is to go downward which philosophically represents the tendency towards gross manifestation. This type of triangle is known as Sakti kona.

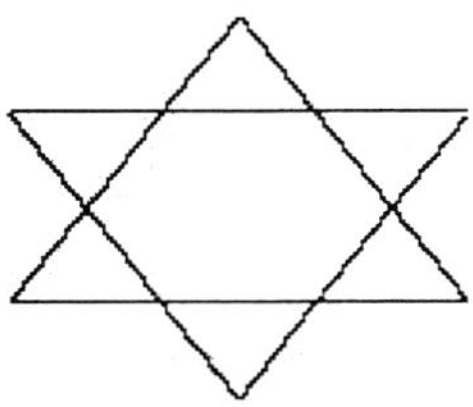

From the combination of these two triangles arises a figure of Satkona or the star with six angles. This figure symbolically represents the union of pururs a-prakriti or Siva-Sakti, without which the creation can not take place. So Satkona is a symbolic representation of the creation of universe.

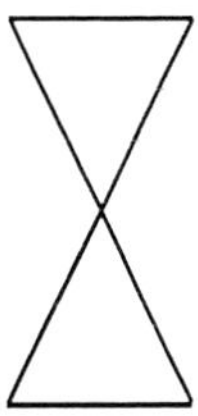

Now let us see how the destruction aspect is symbolized.

This figure like drum of Siva (Damaru) reflects the separation of the union which means the end of creation or destruction or periodic dissolution of cosmos.

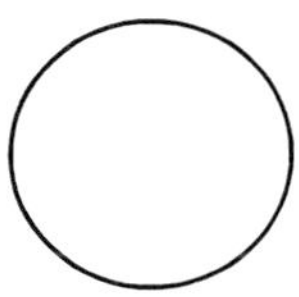

d. Circle:

Triangle expands in the form of circle. Circle represents rotation. It also symbolically presents the air element or vayu tattva. Moreover, it is also an emblem of perfection.

e. Square: Bhùpura:

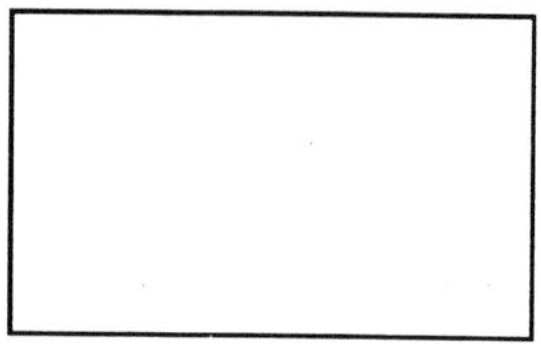

Generally, square is drawn at the outer most limit of the Yantra. It symbolically represents the grossness, which is the quality of the Earth element or the prithvitattva. This figure in Yantra is known as Bhùpura.

Every Yantra starts from Bindu or dot and ends into square or Bhùpura. This shows the process of evolution from subtle to gross, or from ether to earth. Heinrich, Zimmer has very beautifully reflected this view, "On one hand the dynamic diagrams suggests a continuous process of expansion from the centre of the pattern to the circumference and requiring a passage for time for its course. On the other hand they are to be grasped as an enduring hierarchy as gradation of simultaneously manifested degrees of being with the highest value situated at the centre."[10] Danielou, Alain has summarized these figures as a representation of the divinities. We close this point with his view. As he declares, "All the elementary geometrical figures point, straight line, cross, circle, triangle etc. have a symbolical value corresponding to basic notions. They can be combined in more or less complex figures to become the representation of particular force or qualities embodied in some aspect of creation. There is no shape, no movement which may not be reduced to a combination of these elemental forms. The magic diagrams constructed with their help truely analyze and represent the creative force of the cosmos which we call divinities."[11]

There are many types of Yantras meant for securing one or the other objectives like liberation, perfect health, wealth, power, prestige, to overcome diseases, to secure long life etc. The powers cultivated thus are very often used for negative purposes due to human weakness or frailties. They are known as subjugation, attraction, immobilization, dissention, liquidation, cradication and pacification.*

Among Yantras, meant for cultivating highest powers of body-mind for positive purposes beneficial to one's own self as well as for others including animals and subhuman species, Sri Yantra occupies the central place. It is known as king of all Yantras (Yantra Ràja Yantra) because any of the above powers can be cultivated by concentrating on one or more triangle etc. Because of this greatness of the Sri Yantra, we shall see about it in detail.

2. The meaning of Sri Yantra:

Etymologically, Sri is prefix which denotes auspiciousness. Sri Yantra is devised for many purposes shown above and hence its construction is very complex. We shall deal with that aspect in detail later on. For the time being, we should note that the ultimate object of sàdhaka is liberation. Liberation from the bonds of physico-mental as well as spiritual ailments. Concentration on some specific angle or triangle yield freedom from diseases. But man is not satisfied with health only. There are other goals which in other walks of life. Sri Yantra is designed in such a manner that it may be used by a person desirous of anything in the world including freedom from diseases, enemies etc.

This Sri Yantra is considered as the abode of Lalita, the Tàntric name of the Hihger Reality, therefore, it is considered very potent and celebrated among the Yantras.

The emergence of the Sri Yantra is very fascinating. There are various stories regrding its emergence. It is said that the Supreme Sakti of Her own will takes the form of universe and looks at Her own throb with the result that Sri Yantra comes into existence.[12]

This Yantra is also known as Viyat cakra.[13] Viyat means space (Akasa). There are two kinds of Àkasas. The outer space (Bàhyàkàsa) and the inner space (Daharàkàsa).

The outer space is spread over the entire cosmos. And the same again is encapsulated into human body known as inner space or Daharàkàsa. Daharàkàsa, therefore is the same akasa a spread over outside.

The Higher Reality in its evolving process, according to Indian ontology, first manifests in the form of Àkàsa. Àkàsa, therefore, is a visible form of the Higher Reality, as otherwise, Higher Reality being formless is not accessible. Tantra concentrates on the visible manifested from of Higher Reality.

As outer and inner space is identical, sàdhaka by concentrating on inner space, seeks his identity with the Higher Reality. The inner space is the real space for sàdhaka because the Higher Reality resides in the form of space in inner space. Sri Yantra is again a symbol of Daharàkàsa or Higher Reality within.

It is the significant aspect of Sri Yantra that its formation reflects both microcosm and macrocosm. Meditation on it results into realization of the identity between these two.

(i) *Formlation of Sri Yantra:*

Sri Yantra is drawn around a Bindu or dot which is considered as the abode of Lalità, the universal energy. It is described as consisting of super imposition of nine triangles, four with upward apex and five with downward apex. The combination of both produce forty-three triangles. Around these triangles, there are two circles one within the second which contains eight petals while the outer contains sixteen petals. Outside these petals there are three circles and these three circles are covered by the squares known as Bhùpuras. This is the geometrical formation representation of Sri Yantra. Now let us see what it represents symbolically.

(ii) *Symbolic representation of Sri Yantra:*

Sri Yantra starts from Bindu and ends into Bhùpura. It means, in terms of elemental forces, it covers everthing from ether to earth. This shows the way of creation. Between Bindu and Bhùprura, the whole yantra space is divided into three fold and nine fold division as shown below:

The centre of the triangle is known as abode of Lalità. The apex is known as the residence place of Kàmesvari while the left and the right angle are considered as the abiding place of Vajresvari and

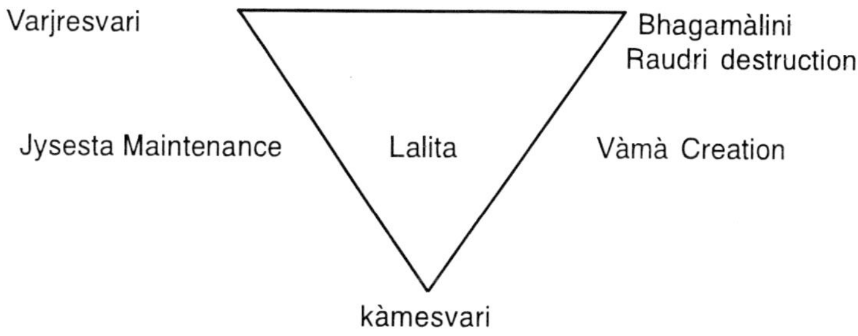

Bhagamàlini respectively. Symbolically, these three deities represent Moon, Fire and Sun respectively. Again, it is also a representation of creation, maintenance and destruction.

(iii) ***Nine fold division:***

The same three fold division from the point of view of gun as becomes nine fold.

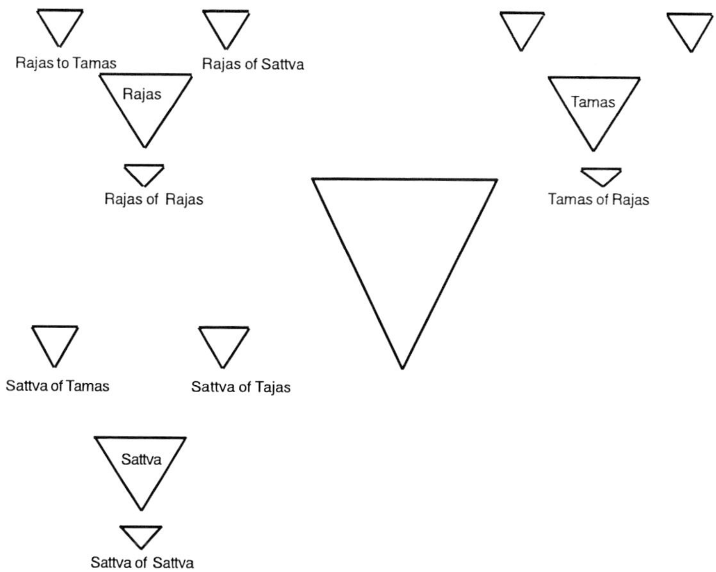

The Sakti or nature in its subtle form is composed of three gunàs, Sattva, Rajas and Tamas. These three gunàs in their active form are convertible to each other. Therefore, the whole division becomes nine fold. Here in the case of gunàs, it is Sattva of Sattva, Sattva of Rajas and Sattva of Tamas. Same is the case with Rajas and Tamas. Thus nine fold division take place.

Between Bindu and Bhùpura, figures like dot, circle, triangle, square take place. They also contain symbolic meaning. Bindu or dot is the centre where creator and creation are in direct contact or identical. Circle represents perfection while square presents grossness. Triangle is an emblem of yoni, a female generative organ or a source of creation.

The Tripuratàpini upanisad has considered triangle as Tripura. Tri means three while pura means abiding place. It is an abiding place of three worlds, namely, earth, heaven and nether world.[14] According to the Tripuropanisad.

Triangle represent gross, subtle and causal aspects both in individual and in cosmic form.[15]

After having seen about the symbolic meanings of the geometrical figure of Sri Yantra, now let us see Sri yantra as symbolical representation of human body.

C. Sri Yantra as symbolic presentation of human body:

Tantra considers body as a temple of divinity. All limbs of body belong to the universal power. These powers representing the limbs of body can be located in Sri Yantra. So Sri Yantra represents the union of body and universe in identity. The significant point is that mere knowledge about this does not help sàdhaka without identifying himself with it by Bhàvanà or imagination. How this identity takes place that we shall see in the words of S. Shankaranarayanan, "The method of arriving at the identity is by offering these members of the human body to the Saktis to whom they originally belonged to the universal powers located in the Sri Cakra. This has to be achieved by Bhavana deep meditation contemplating step by step the various psychophysical parts in the human body and the corresponding powers in the Sri Cakra and dwelling on their identity."[16]

Now we shall see with the help of the figures how physical body is represented in Sri Yantra from Bindu to Bhupura.

Physical body as represented in Sri Cakra:

As we have seen Sri Cakra represents both macrocosm and microcosm. That way it is a link or medium through which one can realize the identity betwen the Ultimate Reality and the Self. In the process of identification, according to Tantra, sadhaka has to mentally imagine (Bhàvayet) the identification of human body, with the universal powers from which the body is composed, and which are imaginably represented by various angles, triangles etc. of Sri Yantra. The Bhav-anopanisad a Sàkta upanisad—has mentioned how the different figures of Sri Cakra represents human body. Thus we shall see the sybmolic representation of the human body in Sri Cakra with the help of Bhàvanopanisad.

The outer most cakra, which is known as Bhùpura contains three lines. The first line as it is mentioned in the chart 2 represents eight powers namely, minuteness, lightness, greatness, lordship, control, power to have whatever one wants, enjoyment, desire, attainment and accomplishment of all desires.[17] The second line of the Bhùpura represents lust, anger, covetousness, delusion, pride, envy, merit and demerit.[18] In the third line of Bhupura, the six centres of the body, the two Sahasràra one above and the other below and Indra yoni are the nine Saktis situated.[19]

The sixteen petalled lotus represents the five gros elements namely, earth, water, five, air, ether, ten senses, namely , ear, skin, eye, tongue, nose, mouth, foot hand arms, gential and the mind.[20]

The eight petalled lotus is an emblem of faculties of speaking, taking, going, excreting, enjoying, rejecting, accepting and ignoring.[21]

The fourteen cornered figure represents fourteen nadis namely, Alambusa, Kuhuh, visvodari, Vàruni, Hastajihvà, Yasovati, Payasvini, Gandhàri, Pushà, Sankhini, Saraswati, Idà, Pingalà, Susumnà.[22]"

The ten cornered figure is a representation of ten vayus, five main and five auxiliary of body namely, Pràna, Apàna, Vyàna, Udàna, Samàna, Nàga, Kurma, Krkara, Devadatta, Dhanañjaya.[23]

The ten breaths acting on the digestive fire of the stomach jatharàigni become tenfold and digest food of all kinds are represented in the ten cornered figure.[24]

The eight cornered figure represents cold, heat, pleasure, pain, wish, sattva, rajas and tamas.[25]

Avyakta, the unmanifest, Mahat the vast cosmic principle force and Ahamkàra the divisional principle of Ego-formation are the three deities in the primary triangle, kàmeswari, Vajreswari and Bhagamalini.[26]

The centre of the Yantra represents the supreme deity Lalita the absolute Reality comprised of Existence-Consciousness Bliss.[27]

Thus Sri Yantra exhaustsal almost all that the Reality contains and hence is the most perfect symbolic representation of Ultimate Reality. It is therefore used in all auspicious ceremonies of Hindu rites. It is also used for protecting the sàdhaka from all evils. Not only this, with the help of Sri Yantra sàdhaka can obtain or master powers of healing, curing diseases and also for driving away evil spirits. Thus it is of tremendous therapeutic value. Wherever such siddha Yantra is kept the house or the place is secured against all evil forces.

3. Therapeutic aspect of Yantra:

Tantra means liberation. It's a process which liberates the sàdhaka from physical-mental and spiritual ailments. Yantra is an aid in Tantra, which enhances this process of liberation.

As Yantra represents human body, the bodily centres or cakras can also be located in Yantras, especially in Sri Yantra. One of the cakras, in sri Yantra, is known as Sarvarogahara cakra or remover of all diseases. Concentration on this centre makes body devoid of diseases. Their therapeutic value has been already mentioned in the

Kundalinì chapter.

Besides this, the Tàntric treatise like Saundrya Lahari, Kalapacintàmanih also refer some Yantras for removing diseases like fever, diabetes, rheumatism etc.*

The Yantras meant for various purposes do not themselves become efficacious. Their efficacy depends upon the effort put in by sadhàka. Yantra is to be worshipped according to certain procedure laid down in the texts like Kalpacintàmanih, Mantra Mahodadhi etc. The entire process is very elaborate and demands astute discipline, concentration as well as observance of certain vows like celiebacy, truth speaking, non-violence, non-attachments etc. Sàdhaka is required to practice all these relentlessness with single minded devotion and unflinching effort. He has to practice fearlessness for sometimes he comes across such experiences which are very much bewildering. It is there fore advised that he should pursue his goals under the guidance of an expert.

The Yantra or Mantra becomes siddha at the end of this elaborate process sometimes lasting for years together but at the end of which the sàdhaka becomes possessed of supernormal powers which help him in helping others for overcoming the ills both physical Psychical as well as spiritual.

In Aserian civilization the entire population practiced drugless therapy for more than 5,000 years. In our country also, there are people existant who claim to cure various diseases with the help of Mantra and Yantra. It is now time we must undertake to examine the possibility to overcome disease by drugless therapies because practice of drugs is getting day-by-day not only irrelevant but also dangerous.

4. Conclusion:

The term 'Yantra' indicates two meanings. One is to control while the second is an instrument. Hence, Yantra is an instrument for gaining control over mental modifications which are considered as the cause of physico mental and spiritual ailments.

In yogic and Tàntric treatise, the cause of diseases is considered as due to disturbance of the elemental forces in outside world on one hand and, or, in the constituents of body on other hand. The geometrical figures, out of which the Yantra is formed namely, dot, circle, square etc. are symbolic representation of the elemental forces. It is believed that medistcation with Mantra on certain figures of Yantra give health. And because of this one of the cakra of the Sri Yantra is known as Sarvarogahara cakra, remover of all diseases.

Among all Yantras, an emphasis has been laid down on Sri Yantra.. As the term Sri indicates , it means auspiciousness. Healthy body-mind is also among them.

Being a symbolic representation of the elemental forces, Sri Yantra also represents both macrocosm and microcosm. So it proves as a link and also as an instrument for realizing the identity between microcosm and macrocosm.

The process of concentration on the Yantra also cultivates the inner latent powers. Power of resistance against disease is also one of them. That way it works as a protection against disease. This process of concentration also prevents diseases by controlling the mental modifications.

The tremendous powers of mind are being wasted in the form of mental modifications. Concentration on Yantra channelize these powers. These channelized powers can be used positively as auto-suggestion in the field of therapy. The disease like insomnia, scrizophenia and other psyco-somatic diseases can be cured by the auto-suggestion therapy.

We have also made reference to Yantras from the Tàntric treatise like Saundrya Laharì and Kalpacintàmanih. The significant aspect, which should not be over looked here. Is that mere Yantra or figure does not give desired results. The latent power of it should be awakened or charged. Especially, in the case of healing, the efficiency of Yantra, depends upon the charging of Yantra done by healer. Though it is a difficult process but at at the same time devoid of any drastic side effects which is very valuable from the therapeutic aspect of Yantra.

Appendix:

1. Yantra from Saundrya Laharì:

The Yantras, which are used for therapy purpose, given below are taken from the Saundrya Lahari of Sri Samkaràcarya.

In the notes under appendix of the Saundrya Laharì, it is written like this: "No originality is claimed for the facts published in this prayoga section. The prayoga should be handled only by those who possess the deserving qualifications and after getting instructions from preceptors or Sri Vidyà upasaka."

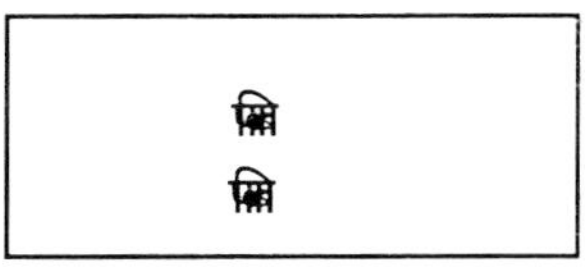

***Prayoga* 12**

Yantra on water or honey placed in silver vessel. Recital 1,000 times for 45 (48) days, facing North-East.

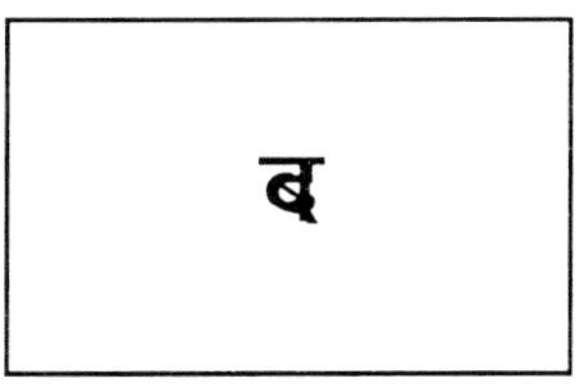

Arcana : Sarasvati, astotara with white flowers and Lalita asototara with jasmine flowers.

Offerings : Cooked rice, pomograntes, honey.

Effects : dumbness cured, power of eloquent speech, gift of poesy.

Prayoga 52

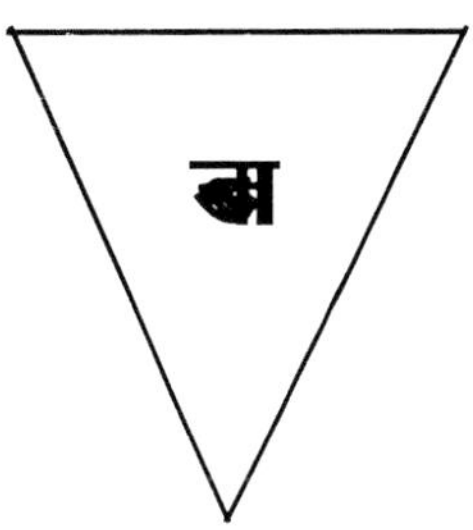

Yantra or goldplate or holy ashes, Recital 10001 times (1000). For 45 days. Facing North-East Archana. Rudrathrisathi with bilva on right side of Yantra and Lalitha-thrisathi with red flowers on left side.

Offering : Cooked rice mixed with sesamum powder, milk-gruel, coconuts and plantains.

Effects : All ear and eye disease cured.

Prayoga 89

Yantra on goldplate or holy ashes. Recital 1008 times for 30 days, facing East. Archanalalitha ashtothara with red flowers.

Offerings : Cooked rice (mixed with curd), sweet-gruel, honey and water.

Effects : Cure of all diseases, physical strength.

2. Yantras from Kalpacintàmanih:

Pacification 1

Name : Jvara-Vinàsanam

Object : Pacifying fever

Description : Draw a yantra with straight lines on all sides and join them. Then draw a quadrangle upon this yantra with eight petals. The yantra should be drawn with the liquid of dhattùrà plant, on a piece of cloth from the dead man's coffin on the spot where the dead are cremated. Thus should be done either on the eight or on the fourteenth day of the dark fornight. Write the name of the person in centre with ram on each of the four sides with ram in each of the eight petals. Worship the yantra by offering lovely flowers collected for the purpose. The process lets even deadly fever disappear immediately.

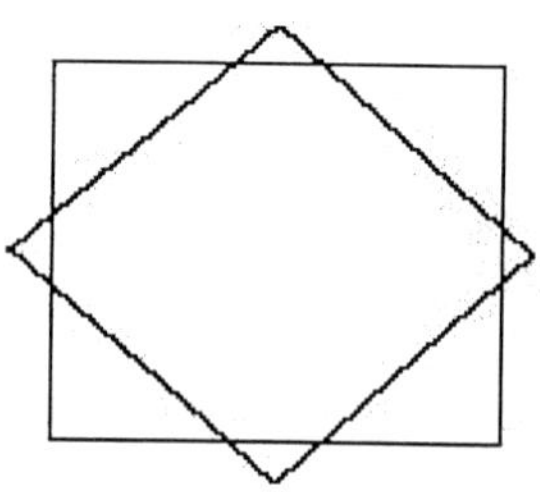

Pacification 13

Name : Sàkini-Dàkini raksàkaram

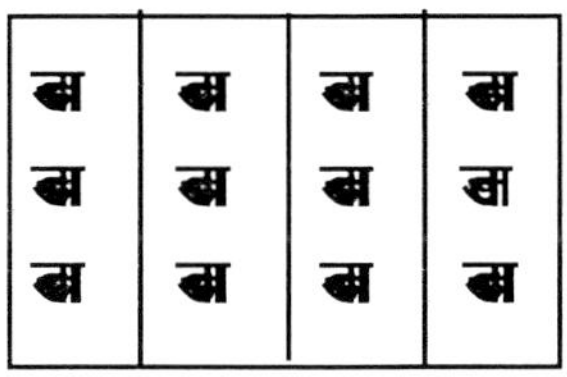

Object : Protecting from evil spirit

Description : Draw this Yantra on a piece of cloth spread over a board but not on the ground. Draw four lines vertically and four horizontally making eight abodes thereby, write ** in each abode and worship the same. Offer presents (bali), flowers, incense, burning candles and drink. Worshipped in this way, the yantra never fails in its aim.*

B. Therapeutic aspect of Mantra :

Introduction

Name and Form are the two inter woven aspects pervading the whole universe. Because of their all pervading nature, they can be the instrument for the realization of Reality. In Tantra, these instruments have been accepted in the form of Mantra and Yantra.

Realization of Reality is nothing but the realization of the original nature of one's own self. This self is like a deity which resides in a temple of body. For getting nearer the deity., one has to cross the gates of body-mind by removing the obstacles through a process of purification and thereby perfecting the body-mind. For this process of purification and perfection, the Mantra and Yantra; one relating to Name and the other relating to Form are, according to Tantra, principal aids. How Yantra purifies body-mind that we have seen under the title "Therapeutic Aspect of Yantra."

Like Yantra, Mantra also works as therapy. Apparently, a Mantra looks like a mere collection of words. And being so a possible question may arise here is that does mere pronunciation of Mantra can cure disease ? The answer is positive provided the words are pronounced according to certain conditions laid down by those who have practiced them and tested their truth. The potency or efficacy of words pronounced by an expert or siddha does not reside in words only. It resides in the efforts of siddha which the word is charged with e.g. The Kuran , The Bible, The Vedas and other holy words.

Here in this chapter an attempt has been made to expose the sound principle on which Mantra therapy stands. We shall proceed first with the meanings of Mantra.

1. Meanings of Mantra:

Human mind can not conceive the nameless and formless Reality. Energies or the Higher Reality, which we call as deities can be reached through symbols like name and form. Only through name and form one can reach nameless and formless. These two symbols are technically called in Tanra, as Mantra and Yantra.

Like Yantra, Mantra also represents deity. The power of deity is inherent in Mantra if it is charged and being so mantras are very powerful and effective. These powers are latent in a Mantra as tree in a seed. A sprout from a seed emerges out only when it gets proper sunlight, water etc. Like wise the latent power of Mantra can be activated by constant repetition, austerity, faith.

The term Mantra is a combination of two terms namely man+tràna. Man means to think or to meditate while tràna means liberation. So in terms of Tantra, we can say, the Sakti which liberates through meditation is Mantra.[1]

Liberation from what ? Liberation of Mind from its various modifications. As we know, mind is very fleeting. It constantly issues various modifications. Due to its fleeting nature it dissipates its energy. If we can prevent his dissipation of energy, or in other terms, if the powers of mind are channelized, they can create such a higher level of mind which is generally not present in lay man. Mantra does this job easily. The concentrated mind is the source of all success. Mantra, therefore, can be one of the most effective instruments for the fulfillment of desires.

Mantras are written in lettters or sabda and can be pronounced with the help of sound. So different sounds contain different types of energy or deity. And because of this proper pronounciation of Mantra is highly required for attainment of gaol. The red light against improper pronounciation of Mantra has been shown by Das gupta, Sasibhusana. As he declares, "...slightest devotion either in articulation or accent or modulation was calculated not only to make them negatively fruitless but positively harmful."[2] By the proper pronounciation of Mantra, as described by Sàstra, controls the energy inherent in Mantra through which he gains whatever he wants. It is not a mere accident but a sound scientific reason lies behind this achievement.

The whole Mantra Sastra is based upon the potentialities of words or sabda. Five gross elements are the constituents of both microcosm and macaroscos, namely Àkàsa, Vàyu, Teja, Àpa and Prithivi. Their origination is stressed back to sabda, sparsa, Rupa, Rasa and Gandha respectively. In this order of creation, Àkàsa, in the gross element, and sabda in the essence of element are considered as most subtle element. The subtlety of sabda is considered to that extent, it is viewed as Brahman or Sabda brahman, source of creation.[3]

Mantras are the collection rather the systematically arranged word-patterns which are very powerful. When a word is pronounced, even at mental level, it creates vibrations. These vibrations throw out from the mind and attract same type of vibrations. Then it becomes a collocation of vibrations when it returns back to its centre, the mind. When it comes back, it becomes more powerful and potential. And becasue of this, if suppose, we want to be good or pure, we should meditate upon such qualities. Constant meditation on particular concept becomes the part of personality.

Though Mantras are powerful but haphazard pronoun-ciations of it does not give any result. In Tantra, certain rules and regulations are prescribed even for the correct pronunciation and recitation of Mantra. A Mantra works only when it becomes realized (Siddha Mantra). A Mantra can not be easily realized . For Mantra sadhana guru or guide is required. First, guru has to decide the

Mantra according to the tendency of sadhaka. In the Sàrdà Tilaka (petal-2) it is declared that if Mantra and sàdhaka, both are in friendly relation, Mantra gives quick results. If the relation between them is of enemy, result is doubtful. A special chart, that is A-Ka-Tha-Ha cakra has been given by Tantra to decide the relationship between sàdhaka and Mantra.

After the selection of Mantra, it should be constantly mentally pronounced with spiritual fervour. He has to assume an yogic posture, perform Nàdi Sodhana, prànàyàma, turn pràna on the way to Susumna and repeat the Mantra when prana flows into Susumna. Austerity Firm faith and devotion in Mantra are also the basic requirements for Mantra siddhi. These are all keys which open the closed doors of treasure of powers.

There are different Mantras prescribed by Tantra, for different purposes. Some of them are give in the appendix.

2. Bija Mantra : Seed Letters :

As tree lies in a seeds, in the same way the power of Mantra lies potentially in a seed letter or bìja mantra. As a tree comes out from seed, likewise the whole Mantra evolves from seed letter. And being so, the seed letters are considered as Yoni, source of creation. Different seed letters are prescribed for different deities. Here we shall see some of them.

1. Seed of speech (vàg-bìja)

Sound : AIM

Definition : This Mantra is also called Sàrasvati (pertaining to knowledge) or Sarasvati (pertaining to the goddess of knowledge). It represents the form of consciousness embodied in the goddess Sarasvati, "Ai represents Sarasvati. The nasalization means the removing of pain. This is the seed-utterance of Sarasvati with it the 'word' is worshipped."

Purpose: Acquiring knowledge and wisdom, mastery over words and power of speech.

Reference: Tripurà tàpini upnisad, Karpura stava and Varadà Tantra.

2. The seed-of-Illusion (màyà bìja) or Seed-of-Energy (Sakti bìja)

Sound: HRIM

Definition: This Mantra represents màyà the power of illusion. It stands for the lady-of-spheres (Bhuvanesvari), the dispeller of sorrow. It is root from which develop ether and other elements of the manifest world, the principle over liberated, unbounded by the triple form of time. "Ha means Siva. R is his Nature Prakriti. I means Transcendent Illusion (mahà-màyà). The sound is the progenitor of the universe. The nasalization means the removing of sorrow. The lady of the sphere should be worshipped with this (Mantra) (Varadà Tantra).

Purpose: Conquest of the unmanifest, of the power of Nature. Transgressing the laws of time and space.

Reference: Tripurà tàpini upnisad 1. 13 Karpura Stava, Varadà Tantra etc.

3. The seed-of-Existence or Seed-of-Fortune (laksmì-bìja)

Sound: SRIM

Definition: This mantra represents the goddness of fortune and multiplicity, Laksmì, the consort of Vishnu. 'S' represents the transcendent divinity of fortune. R means wealth. Ì is satisfaction. The sound means 'limitlessness'. The nasal-ization means the dispelling of sorrow. This is the seed utterance of the goddess Lakshmì through which she should be worshipped." (Varadà Tantra)..

Purpose: Gaining worldly wealth, power, beauty and glory.

Reference: Tripura tàpini upanisad, Varadà Tantra etc.

4. The Seed-of-Desire: (kàma-bìja)

Sound: KLIM

Definition: This mantra represents the form of joy of pleasure, the procreative aspect of the power of Siva in the form of his consort, the Transcendent-Goddess (Mahesvari). 'K' represents Eros. (kàmadeva) or Krsna, the incarnation of divine lust. L means the lord of heaven Indra. I means satisfaction. The nasalization is the giver of both pleasure and pain. The seed of Desire is spoken to you out of love, O Great Goddess." (Varadà Tantra).

Purpose: Gaining transcendent knowledge and also pleasure, victory and royal power.

Reference: Tripurà tàpini upnishad, Karpura stava, Varadà Tantra.

5. The Primordal-Seed (àdyà-bìja) or seed-of-the-Power-of Time (Kàlì-bija):

Sound: KRIM

Definition: This mantra represents the power of time, the power of death, the destructive aspect of Siva and thus the goddess Kàlì, the power of time.

'K' is Kàlì. R is the Brahman. I is the transcendent power of illusion. The sound is the "Mother of the Universe". The nasalization is the dispelling of sorrow. The goddess Kàlì should be worshipped with this mantra to the pacifying of all pain." (Varadà Tantra)

Purpose: Gaining detachment power over death transcendent knowledge.

References: Tripurà tapini upnisad, Mahànirvàna and Varadà Tantra.[4]

Other seed letters

Dum	-	Durgà
Gam	-	Ganapati
PHAT	-	Weapon for destroying anything
STRÌM	-	Liberates from difficulties

Seed letters of the Elements:

LAM	-	Earth-Prithvi
VAM	-	Àp. water
RAM	-	Teja-Fire
YAM	-	Vàyu-Air
HAM	-	Àkash -Ether

The Thought-Form of Fifteen Syllables (Pancadasi) of the first Goddess:

Test — Ka-e-i-la-hrim, Ha-sa-ka-ha-la-hrim,
Sa-ka-la-hrim.

Meaning:

Ka	-	lust
e	-	womb (or speech)
i	-	the substance of lust
la	-	thunder bolt-bearer (or the earth, or Siva)
hrim	-	a cave (the seed mantra of the Goddess).
ha	-	Siva
Sa	-	energy
Ka	-	Wind (or lust)
la	-	Lord of heaven (Indra) or Siva
ha	-	cloud (or Siva)

Definition: this represents the power of the self, the power of enchantment of the world.

No. of repetition: to be repeated twenty one or 108 times.

Purposes: to attain all the desires and liberation.

Reference: Devi upnishad Nityà soda-Sikàrnava, Varivasyà Rahanya etc.[5]

These Bija mantras should be constantly repeated for quick results. The process of constant repetition is known as japa. Now we shall see something about japa.

C. Japa:

Japa sàdhanà is prescribed by all religious. It plays significant role in sadhana. Because of its significance, Lord Krishna had declared, 'I am the japa yajna, among all yajnas. (Yajña, among all yajnas. (Yajñànàm japayajñosmi II)

Japta is a spiritual exercise. It is a scientific process for cultivation of will power. Mantra japa ensures various powers which is also again helpful in coming over the hurdles lying in the way of success.

How japa does this work or what is the meaning of japa this can be asked. In the term japa, 'Ja' removes the vicious circle of life and death while 'pa' removes sins. Hence japa is that which removes both the circle of life and death and also sin.[6] There are various ways designed by Tantra for the repetion of Mantra or japa. These various ways we shall see uner the title "Kinds of japa".

1. Kinds of Japa:

1. Nitya japa:

As bathing, eating etc. are required for the maintenance and purification of external body likewise, for the internal purification, mental exercise like japa is required. This should be done daily without any exception.

2. Kàmya japa:

Japa is done for various purposes. The japa which is done for the fulfillment of specific desire, it is known as Kàmya japa.

3. Acala japa:

Japa sàdhanà varies according to the goal of desire. A number of japa is fixed which should be compulsorily be done for the attainment of the desired goal. This type of japa also should be done at fixed place and time. This process strengthens the will power of sàdhaka which ultimately results into success.

4. Cala japa:

Cala japa can be done at any time or in any situation. No rules and regulations are prescribed for this. The nature of mind is to think either good or bad. For avoiding the bad thoughts this cala japs is utilized.

5. Vàcika japa:

Japa which is done in loud voice is known as Vàcika japa. this type of japa is considered at low and works only at initial level of sàdhanà. Though it is considered as low, it is good for concentration of mind.

6. Upànus japa:

In this type of japa, only the movement of lips takes place but no sound is heard. This type of japa helps in the internalization of sense which are generally externalized.

7. Mànsika japa:

In this type of japa, neither tongue nor the movement of lips takes place. It is done only at mental level. Because of its substicity, it is considered as the best type of japa.

8. Ajapà japa:

This type of japa is done without màlà. This should be done with the process of respiration. While exhalation, Mantra Ham and while inhalation, Mantra Sah should be pronounced.

All these types of japa differ only in the manner of pronounciation. The basic principle of japa sàhdanà is that it should be done constantly with faith, devotion and concentration.

2. Therapeutic Aspect of Japa:

Japa means constant mediation on specific concept. It is the nature of mind that the idea on which it constantly medaites becomes the part of personality. It we think positively, mind also becomes positive which impact also can be felt on body. Negative thinking harms both body and mind. This necessarily leads us to infer that mediation on idea of good health invariably results into good health.

Mental tension is the root of most of the diseases. In this age of fast life, we constautly have to face mental tensions. By constant repetition of Mantra, mind togets everything about the external world and that way mind gets relief from tensions.

Japa also increases faith in God. God is omnipotent and whatever happens, it happens either for good or for bad is due to his wish. So there is no reason to be worried about anything. Tranquilliozers and drugs like campose also do this job, In fact actually doing more harm to the body than good. Japa, therefore is an innocent and yet psychologically better, longtime lasting remedy than any type of tranquillizers.

D. Therapeutic aspect of Mantra:

Till now, Mantra has been considered as mere hypocrisy and humbug. But now it has been accepted scientifically, specially in the area of therapy, or as a healing agency.

The connotation of the term Mantra itself shows that it liberates its sadhaka (Mananàttrànàt iti Mantra). It liberates its sàdhaka from physico-mental-spiritual troubles). (Adhi-Vyàdhi-Upàdhi) Mental troubles like tension generated from the complexities of life. the possessor of the worried mind becomes unhappy and ultimately becomes a victim of mental disease like scrizophenia, split personality etc.

The intense form of tension end into the psychosomatic diseases. It makes both body-mind diseased. Mantra japa makes one free from worries and that why it also removes the bonds of mental physical disorders.

There are certain reasons which are considered as the cause of disease. One of them is the imbalance of hormonal secretions of lands. Over secretions and under secretions both create disorder in body-mind. Proper secretions depend upon mental state of a person. When a person is in a happy mood, glands do not work properly. While if mind is not in a happy mood, glands do not work properly. This improper way of working of glands results into disease. Mantra gives happiness to mind and keeps mind silent. In the silent mind glands work without any obstacles or disturbances and that way here, Mantra works indirectly as therapy.

The impact of Mantra japa also can be seen on the brain cells. Our brain is divided into two halves. The large brain and the small brain. The small brain contains a portion known as hypothelamus. In this area of brain, cells of hunger, thirst etc.. are located. When a person is under tension he becomes more excited which results into high blood pressure. It has been worked out that constant repetition of Mantra japa decreases this excitement and also normalize the blood pressure.

How Mantra does this job? Mantra therby is largely related with the process of autosuggestion mentioned by Psychology, in which either healer or a patient has to give a constant suggestion. Here, in the Mantra therapy, constant repetition of Mantra or letters, penetrates the conscious mind and the sound waves of Mantra enters into the subconscious mind is more powerful than conscious mind, and its impact also can be seen on the body-mind. So the impact of positive state of subconscious mind effects body-mind positively. This positively can be induced by Mantra japa.

In the healing through Mantra, by constant of repetition of Mantra, sàdaka concentrates his mind on a Mantra which produce a state of tranquillity.[6] So this state of meditation. This state of meditation works as therapy in two ways. Firstly, meditation makes man aloof from the external mental tension which are considered as the root of diseases and secondly, the state of meditation is a result of concentrated mind. This cultivates inner latent will power or the power of resistance against diseases. Thus by removing the mental tensions and by cultivating inner power, meditation works as therapy. Mantra-japa is the easiest and the best way for inducing such a state of meditation.

The healing through Mantra is possible by two ways. One is self healing while in second type of healing, heal heals patient. In a diseased body, it is not always possible to do Mantra. In such a case, a Mantra healer transfers his inner power into a patient. Here letters of Mantra work like channel through which power travels. The permanence of the cure done by Mantra, depends upon the intensity of the inner power of a healer.

The concept of the Màntric therapy also has been accepted by the Àyurveda, an Indian art of meditation. The seers of Ayurveda, Caraka and Susruta have accepted it as therapy.[7]

Besides this, Mantra therapy is also utilized for removing the poison. Sueruta has mentioned the process of removing the poison by Mantra in the kalpasthàna of his samhità. "A physician well versed in the Mantras of antivenomous potency should bind a leigature of a cord consecrated with appropriate Mantras which would arrest a further spread of the poison. The Mantras full of occult energy of perfect truth and divine communion, disclosed by the Devarshis and Brahmins of yore, never fail to eliminate the poison from the system, and hold their own even in the case of deadliest poisons".[8]

There are also some Mantras, prescribed by Tantra for health and longlife which are here, given in the appendix.

In the Mantric thereapy, there is nothing like miracle of humbug. It is just a way of cultivation of inner resistance power against diseases and positively strengthening the will power in the case of self-healing while in the case of healer and patient, a sàdhaka who has realized the Mantra, transfers his awakened powers through the medium of Mantra.

In the concluding portion of this chapter, we can say that., Mantra and Yantra are the two aids of Tantra. Tantra has penerated the very root of disease, that is, unbalanced mind. Mantra and the Yantra are the instruments through which one can stabilize the mind. This stabilized or concentrated become full proof against all kinds of external attacks of diseases.

Appendix:

3. Mantras prescribed by Tantra for different purposes:

1. Remover of diseases:

Aum sam sàm sim sìm sum sùm sem saum sam sah

vam vàm vim vìm vùm vem vaim voum vah vah

ham sah amruta varcase svàhà

— Uddisi Tantra

2. Bestower of liberation (Moksa):

Srìm hrìm krìm krusnàya namah

— Gautamiya Tantra

3. Giver of Dharma, Artha, Kama and Moksa:

Aum saccideka brahma-

— Mahanirvàna Tantra

These mantras are taken from the Tantra Mahàvijñàn by Sri Rama

Sarma, pp. 454-55.

4. Mantras for health and long life:

In the eleventh chapter of the Durga Saptasati, there is a verse in which sàdhaka asks to devi for health.

Rogànasesànapahamsiustà rustà tu kàmàn sayalanàbhisàana II

In the Argalà stotra of Devi stuti, it is also asked to devi for health.

Delhi Saubhàgyamàrogyam dehi devi paramam sukham

— Argalà stotra, 12

A mantra for long life is prescribed into the Rudràstàdhyàyi.

Aum trayambakam yajàmahe sugandhimpusti vardhanamII

Urvàrùikamive bandhanàt mrutyo mukhiyamamrutàt II

— Rudràstàdhyàyi, 515

CHAPTER - 7

THERAPEUTIC ASPECT OF TANTRA

CHAPTER - 7

1. Introduction:

Desired life span or a long life has always been a matter of attraction of the human race. Tantra has its own unique method of healing and for prolonging life span.

Tantra has penetrated the very root of disease. It removes the accumlation of impurities which is also one of the causes of disease from the body vessels and also from subtle channels. It purifies the body vessels through the six purificatory actions (satkriyàs) mentioned by the Hathayoga. While it removes the impurities of subtle channels through the process of Sumanu described by the Gherand Samhità. The process of the Bhuta Suddhi, the important aspect of Tantra sàdhanà also plays an important role in the purification of body-mind complex.

Moreover, Tantra has also mentioned the process of streightening the purified body through the intake of the Rasa or prepared mercury (pàrada).

These processes largely deal with the purification of body. It has also mentioned certain techniques through which, the body which has already become a victim of disease can be cured. The unique methods of Tàntric healing are the Science of breathing known as Siva Swarodays, Mudrà, process of Sat karma, Mantra, Yantra etc. Among all these we have already dealt in detail about Mantra and Yantra therapy. In this chapter we shall try to focus the Tantric way of rejuveration and various kinds of healing. Let us proceed with the purification of physical body.

2. Purification of Physical Body:

In Tàntrism, human body enjoys significant place. As the Gheranda Sambhità (1.8) declares, the body is no longer a source of pain, but the most reliable and effective instrument at man's disposal for "conquering death". And science liberation can be gained even in this life, the body must be preserved as long as possible and in perfect condition, precisely as an aid to meditation.[2]

For preserving the body in perfect condition, Tantra especially the Hathayoga, prescribes the method of training and developing the body and mind. The goal of Tantra is to discover the hidden layers of mind, potential powers of body and to awaken the inner spiritual faculties, For this, control over physical body is highly required. In the Hathayoga, control over body starts with the cleaning process known as purificatory actions or kriyàs. They are six in number hence they are known as Sat kriyàs. These actions or processes help in the elimination of the poisonous substance accumulated in the bodily channels.

Accumulation of poison in channels is also one of the causes of disease. Body constantly throws waste materials through urine, perspiration, excretion etc. It constantly does this process. The Hatheyogic purificatory process enhances this process of elimination of waste products of body.

(i) *Hathayogic way of purification of body:*

The sat kriyàs or the six purificatory actions mentioned by the Hathayoga covers the entire body. They are meant for cleaning the respiratory system, *food pipe, eyes, stomach, lower colon* etc.. The name of these kriyàs are *Dhauti, Basti, Neti, Nauli, Tràtaka and kapalabhàti.*[2] These actions clean stomach, colon, nasal passage, abdominal organs, eyes and respiratory organs respectively. We shall proceed first with Dhauti.

a. Dhauti:

Dhauti means washing. It is divided into four types:

1) Internal washing—Antardhauti;

2) Cleaning of teeth—Danta dhauti;

3) Cleaning throat—Hrid dhauti;

4) Cleaning of rectum—Moola Sodhanam.[3]

Again the internal washing, Antardhauti is divided into four parts: (1) Wind purification—Vàtàsàra. (2) Water purification—Varisara, (3) Fire purification— Vahnisaran, (4) Cloth purification—Vastarasàra.

Wind purification: Vàtasàra:

In this process, one should swallow the air to the stomach by closing the epiglottis till the stomach is filed with air. Then move that air therein and then slowly force it out through lower passage.

Water purification: Varisàra:

Drink a large quantity of water to which a little salt is added and then shake the abdominal portion. Then vomit it out by putting finger at the root of the tongue. This should be done in the morning on an empty stomach. This prevents constipation.

Fire purification: Vahnisara:

A person who wants to do this, should sit in a comfortable posture. To perform it, the trunk should bent forward, hands put on the knees and deep inhalation be performed. Hold the breath outside as far as possible. While holding the breath, push the abdomen backward and forward. This process stimulates all the portion with abdomen, viz., stomach, intestine, liver, spleen, pancreas etc. This process removes constipation.

Cloth purification: Vastrasara:

This process prescribes the purification of the limentry canal. This canal is a long tube extended from mouth to anus and covers the area of mouth, pharynx , oesophagus, stomach, large and small intestine.

The cloth purification is prescribed in the following way:

Take a fine piece of cloth, three inches wide and fifteen feet long. No piece of loose thread should be hanging from its side. Wash the piece. Dip it in tepid salt water. Then swallow the one end of it little by little. On the first day swallow it only one foot.

Then increase it by daily practice. During process do not be hasty. This process should be done with empty stomach preferable in the morning. This process is beneficial for the abdominal and respiratory disorders.

2. Danta Dhauti: Cleaning of teeth:

Danta dhauti is massaging of teeth with water or powdered earth so long as dental impurities are not removed.

3. Hrid dhauti: Purification of tongue:

For cleaning the root. Put the three fingers, index, middle and ring, in a joint manner. Rub well the root of the tongue. Wash it again and again. Repeat this process. This process helps in bringing out excretion from stomach and lungs.

4. Moola Sodhanam: Cleaning of rectum:

Moola Sodhanam is a cleaning of rectum. With the help of the middle finger, the rectum should be carefully cleansed with water again and again. This process destroys constipation, indigestion etc.

b. Neti: Nasal Cleaning:

Neti is a cleaning of nasal passage of the respiratory system. There are two types of neti. (1) Suta neti and (2) Jala neti.

In Suta neti, take thin thread and insert it into nostril and passing it through it, pull it out by mouth.

The jala neti can be done with the help of lukewarm salt water. Pour a small portion of the salt water through one nostril by closing the other nostril with thumb. Raise the head and allow the water to flow down to the throat and expel it out through mouth. The remaining portion of the water in the mouth should be blown out by forced expiration.

This process removes disorders of cold and ensures sharp eye sight.

c. Tràtaka:

Trataka is a gazing at particular point without waking the eye. This process can be done by various ways.

In one of the methods, a candle flame is kept three feet away from the person. The flame and the eye should be in a horizontal line. In the comfortable posture, with the spine straight but relaxed position, person looks at the flame for a minute. After that he closes the eyes, relax the eye muscle and visualize that flame between the eyebrows. Again do this process. This may be continued 4 or 5 times. This exercise brings concentration and strengthens eyes.

In other Tràtaka technique, called Bhrumadhya drisit, the half closed eyes are directed upward toward the space between the eyebrows. This process enables the mind to become painted.

In the Nàsàgra dristi, the gazing takes place at the tip of the nose. This process strengthens the eye muscles and increases concentration.

d. Kapàlabhàti:

This is an exercise for the purification of the nasala passage and lungs. This process is specially designed to remove the spasm in bronchial tube. This also helps in curing Asthma and also removes impurities of blood.

Technique:

After assuming a lotus posture, take a few deep breaths. Then rapid inhaltion exhalation should be done. More attention should be given on exhalation. Start one round of this exercise with ten expulsion at the end of the tenth explusion take deep inhalation. Gradually increase the number of rounds.

e. Nauli:

Nauli is an exercise for purification and strengthening the abdominal muscles. Before doing the nauli process, the practice of the Uddiyana bandha—abdominal contraction is necessary.

Technique of Uddiyàna bandha:

Sit in any meditative posutre. One has to empty the links by a strong and forcible expiration. When the lings are empty, the diaphragm raises naturally to the thoracic caviaty. Draw up the intestine and the navel toward back of the body. Keep the abdomen as long as one can hold the breath comfortably outside without inhaling.

Nauli:

The same process of contraction takes place in the nauli kriya. While in Uddiyàna bandha, allow the centre of the abdomen to be free by contracting the left and right side of the abdomen. This is known as Madhya nauli.

After mastering this, the next stage is to control over the left and right muscle of abdomen. This is known as Vama and Daksina nauli.

f. Basti: Cleaning of lower colon:

The basti process of cleaning is done by creating a vacuum through nauli kriyà in the intestine.

Sit in a tub of water and practice nauli. Create vacuum in intestine. To keep the spincter muscle open, insert a small tube about four inches in length into the rectum. As soon as the water is drawn, the tube should be removed. And with a few abdominal churnings (nauli), the water is thrown out from the large intestine with muscles and other waste products.

This process cleanesses the abdominal muscles and cures urinary and digestive disorders.

From the above mentioned description of the six purificatory actions mentioned by the Hathayoga, we can see that, these processes cover the whole body. By applying these processes one can purify one's body, with the result that one can not be the victim of physical diseases.

As we know, the origin of the physical diseases are located in the mental disturbances. So mind also should be purified, or in other terms, should be concentrated. The application of the pranayama technique is the best way for concentration of mind. As the pre-requirement for performing the prànàyàma is a purification of Nadis or channels. As we know, in our body a net of nerves is spread cut. Prana or the vital breath moves through this channels. It there is any impurities in them, it is difficult for prana to move. So first Nàdi purification is required.

Now we shall see how this nàdi purification can be done with the help of the Tàntric seed letters like vam, ram, tham etc.

3. Tantric way of Nàdi purification:

The fifth lesson of the Gherand Samhità declares the Samanu process of purification which should be done mentally with the Bìja-Mantra or seed letters. The translation of the verses runs as follows:

Sitting in the Padmasàna posture, and performing the adoration of the Guru. As taught by the Teacher, let him perform purification of Nàdis for success in pranyama. Contemplating on Vàyu-Bìja (i.e. yam), full of energy and of a smoke colour, let him draw in breath by the left nostril, repeating the Bija sixteen times. This is puràka. Let him restrain the breath for a period of sixty-four repetition of the Mantra. This is Kumbhaka. Then let him expel the air by the right nostril slowly during a period occupied by repeating the Mantra thirty-two times.

The root of the navel is the seat of Agni-tattva. Raising the fire from that place, join the Prithvi-Tattva with it, then contemplate on this mixed light. Then repeating sixteen times the Agani-Bìja (Ram, let him draw in breath by the righ nostril, and retain it for the period of sixty-four repetition of the Mantras, and then expel it by the left nostril for a period of thirty-two repetitions of the Mantra.

Then fixing the gaze on the tip of the nose and contemplating the luminous reflection of the moon there, let him inhale through the left nostril, repeating the Bija (tham) sixteen times; let him retain it by repeating the Bìja (tham) sixty-four times; in the meanwhile imagine (or contemplate) that the nectar flowing from the moon at the tip of the nose runs through all the vessels of the body and purifies them. Thus contemplating, let him expel the air by repeating thirty-two times the Prithvi Bìja lam.

By these three pranayamas the nàdis are purified. Then sitting firmly in a posture let him begin regular prànàyàma.[4]

Thus by applying the Hathayogic way of purification, sàdhaka purifies his bodily vessel, while by applying the Sumanu process, a Tàntric way of purification, sàdhaka purifies subtle channels through which vital air flows. Beyond these two, there is also another Tantric way, that is the purification of body. Bhuta Suddhi, which is the integrated part of Tàntric sàdhanà, which we have already seen in the chapter 'Tàntric sàdhanà'. To avoid the repetition of it, here in a nutshell, we can say that, in the process of the Bhùta Suddhi, sadhaka has to imagine a man of impurities (pàpa purusa) and that man should be first dried out then burnt away mentally. After destroying this man of impurities, sàdhaka has to create a new divine body with the help of the elixir of the Sahasràra cakra. This whole process should be done mentally. While destroying the man of impurities sadhaka destroys bodily impurities and that way this process secures bodily purification.

Purification of body is not the only goal of Tanra but that purified body should be strengthened like rock so that it can resist any kind of physical mental disturbances. For that, Tanra has prescribed the theory of Rasa.

4. Theory of Rasa: A Tantric way of rejuvenation:

The Nàtha siddhas and the Rasa siddhas are the two Tàntric cults which are based on the ideal of liberation during life-time, Jivan-mukti. In order to keep body undecayable many experiments were made by Tàntrics. Among them use of mercury for rejuvenation of body is the main one.

Tantra considers man or human body as the highest evolute of the nature. As such the essence of the cosmic world, it believes, is embodied in human body. The natural deduction of this theory is that, there is nothing in the cosmos which is not there in human body.

The Nàtha cult and the Rasa siddhas believe that the process of evolution has three stages. The creation, the maintenance and the destruction. Absolute Reality is believed to pass through these three stages when the process of manifestation starts. The creation function is symbolically identified with Moon, while destructive function is identified with the Sun. The goal of the Natha siddhas is to attain the non-dual state of immortality. This can be attained by the union of Sun-Moon located inside the body.

According to these two cults, death or decay takes place because the elixir which trickles down from the Moon situate at the Sahasràra, ordinarily falls into the fire of the Sun, which is located at the navel region, where it is dried away. Thus the elixir of body, being dried up the body becomes a victim to the destruction. This is the ordinary course of the flow of nectar which must be checked. The elixir should not be consumed. If once it is done, sàdhaka gets control over time means enjoys desired life span.

Utilization of alchemy (Rasa) is one of the ways of getting control over time. In Sanskrit lexicon, the meaning of this term is juice but in Tàntrism it is specifically used for mercury.

Tàntric alchemical ideas grow around the Siva-Sakti symbolism. Mercury is considered as the male principle or Siva while sulphur is considered as the female principle or Sakti. The substance that is produced through the combination of these two elements makes the creature immortal.[5]

Rasa is called pàrada because it leads one to the other shore of the world.[6] It is also considered as the seed of Siva.[7] This mercury or parade is said to be able to do two extraordinary things: (1) Rejuvenation of body and (2) Conversion of base metal into gold. Here we are concerned only with the first purpose.

Mercury can not be utilized in a naked form dour to its poisonous nature. So for the medicinal use of it, it has to undergo eighteen different processes (Samskàras). This prepared mercury should be utilized as giver of immortality.

This theory of Rasa discloses the secret of the prolonged life of our ancient seers. So by the Hathayogic way of bodily purification, Tàntric way of purification of subtle nerves and by intake of the prepared mercury, one can get control over decay. The basic requirement for all processes is that, at initial level, it requires the guidance of an expert without which instead of long life one can be victim of death.

This is about the purification of body. If suppose somebody becomes victim of disease how he can cure himself we shall see now.

(i) *Various Tàntric ways of healing:*

Tantra not only purifies the body but it also removes the diseases which are already there in the body. There are various ways of this. Among them techniques of Sat kriyàs, Siva sworodaya, Mudra etc. are unique one.

Sat karma is a process followed by contemplation on specific Bìja-Mantra or seed letters like yam, vam, ram etc. Sat karma samgraha is a text of both yoga and àyurveda prescribed by Lord Siva Himself.[8] Now we shall see Sat karma process with the help of the treatise Sat karma samgraha.

A. *Sat karma : Six actions:*

Sat karma, six actions, are six in number which are namely (a) Ùrdhvacakrì, (b) Madhyacakrì, (c) Adhacakrì, (d) Tràtakam, (e) Kasà and (f) Netrìkaranam.[9] We shall explain, in brief, each of them.

a. *Ùrdhvacakrì:*

This process is performed by entering one's own thumb wet with water, in the centre of the palate. Then rotate it. By doing again and again, the impurities, which are situated there can be removed.[10]

As this treatise, Sat karma samgraha, declares while doing this process, he has to contemplate upon the bright triangular Ram, Bìja-Mantra or seed letter of fire. Constant practice of this process removes the impurities of eyes, ears etc.[11]

b. *Madhyacakrì:*

This process is done by inserting the finger at the root of the tongue and the front of the uvula. Rotate the finger there with the remembrance of the god of Agni. By constant practice of this process the excess phlegm can be removed.[12]

c. *Adhacakrì:*

In this, the index finger should be entered in the anus. This process should be continued till the expansion of the anus with the contemplation on Yam seed letter. This process removes dropsy, disease of rectum, enlargement of spleen.[13]

d. *Tràtakam:*

This process is done by the fixation of the eyes on a minute object till tears begin to fall. This should be done without winking the eyes with the repetition of the seed letter of water, that is, Vam. This removes all the diseases of eyes and also sleepiness.[14]

e. *Kasà:*

In this process, a fine smooth thread should be introduced into throat through nose. The friction of the thread in nose and throat removes the disorders of the phlegm.[15]

f. *Netrìkaranam :*

In this process, a clean, soft, strong lubricated made of white thread should be introduced into the Idà and taken out from the pingalà.[16]

Thus the application of the process of Sat kriyà removes the disease like dropsy, sleepiness, disease of ears, eyes, dis-orders of phlegm etc. These processes have a resemblance with the six purificatory actions mentioned by the Hathayoga. It differs on the ground that these process should be done with the repetition of the seed letters while in the Hatheyogic practice, no repetition of Mantra takes place.

There is also one another treatise, like Sat Karma Samgraha, a dialogue between Lord Siva and Pàrvatai, is Siva svarodayam. It's a scripture related with the process of inhalation and exhalation. It has mentioned the technique of diagnosis, the disease by pattern of breathing process and technique of healing by manipulating the breathing process. Now we shall see something about the Svarodays, a science of breathing.

(ii) *Siva Svarodaya: A Science of breathing:*

Siva Svarodaya is a scripture, told by Siva to Parvatia for the welfare of the human beings. This treatise is based on the concept of vital force or pràna sakti which pervades in the entire body. The vital force is the very core of life. This can be seen by the difference between a living body and a dead body. In former, there is a presence of life force or prana sakti while in later it is absent.

In reply to one of the questions of Pàrvati, Lord Siva says, pràna is the best friend and best brother. Nothing is superior to prana. Breathing is the gross form of that vital force or pràna sakti.[17]

Pràna Sakti is related with both body and mind. Physical body is gross while mind is subtle. Pràna is link between these two body mind. Hence it affects both.

The very existence of the physical body as living entity is dependent upon the presence of pràna. This shows the superiority of prana over body. The relation of mind and pràna is also very well known. They are so highly related that as the Hathayoga pradipika declares, by controlling one, the other can be controlled.

Mental disturbances are considered as the root of the disease. This type of disturbances occur due to the fleeting nature of mind. Generally, it is difficult to control the mind but by controlling the vital force, through breathing process, mind can be controlled.

Here the control over breathing process is different from that of the prànàyàma process. As we know, we do inhalation and exhalation either through the right nostril or through the left nostril. Siva Svaroday mentions the duration period of the respiration process which takes in one nostril. At every two hours duration, there is a change in the nostril operating at that time.

We can ascertain which nostril must be working at a particular time during the day and at night. The scripture lays down the correct process of working the nostril at particular time. The working of the opposite nostril shows the imbalance and hence a signal to the disease. The disease can be cured by changing the working of the nostril.

So in this process of healing, disease is diagnized by the working of nostril and healed by the manipulation of it. This therapy is also based on the Tàntric principle of the identical relationship between microcosm and macrocosm.

Physical body is a miniature universe. The sun and a moon which are highly associated with the vital force and mental force respectively can also be located in the body. As we have already mentioned in the chapter of Tantra sàdhanà that, pràna or vital force flows through subtle channels which are spread out like a net in a body. Three are the main channels, namely, Idà, Pingalà and Susumnà. Susumnà is a meru or a spinal cord along with the former two channels run on the left and right side of it respectively.

Sun is located at the right sides and being so the vital current flows throgh the Pingalà nàdi. While moon is located at the left side and hence mental currents flow through Idà nàdi. The flow of breathing through Idà and Piñgalà takes place through the left and right nostril respectively.

By considering these two above mentioned principles on which this therapy is based, we can say that over working under working or mafunctioning of any nostril creates imbalance in mental and vital current. Over working of right nostril, being related with Sun, results in the vigorous personality. While in the case of Idà, being related with Moon, person becomes victim of caprice.

This fact is also noted by the science, that when the right side and left hemisphere is predominant during a particular time one becomes more aggressive. While more passive functions are to be performed when the left side is predominant.

There is also one another way of Tàntric healing which is also based on the principle of identity betwen macrocosm and microcosm. The name of this technique is Mudra or gesture.

(iii) *Mudrà: Gestures:*

Mudrà is an integrated part of daily Tàntric sàdhanà. It is also one of the pañca Makàras which we have already seen in the Tantra symbolism.

Mudrà is a gesture of hand initially but its goal is total mental identification. Mudrà is based on the principle of identity between macroscosm and microcosm.

Like universe, body is also composed of five elements namely earth, water, fire, air and ether. These elements are situated in the body in a fixed proportion. Mudràs are the means to normalize this proportion of the five elements in the body.

It is believe, the control over five gross elements, the constituents of the body, is located at the five fingers of the hand. The thumb represents space, the forefinger wind or air, the middle finger fire, the ring finger water and the fourth finger represents earth.[18] So thus the control over each element is possible through the fingers.

a. *Pràna Mudra:*

Pràna mudrà is designed for curing the disease like heart attack, one of the prominent diseases of this age.

"..... a patient having a heart attack can check the attack and get instant relief by folding the forefinger down on the mound of the thumb, and joining the thumb with the tips of the third and fourth finger.[19]

b. *Sùnya Mudrà:*

"Bend the Madhyàma middle finger, to touch the root of the thumb. Then press it slightly with the thumb.[20] This mudrà removes deafness.

c. ***Sùrya Mudrà:***

Bend the Anàmikà, (the third ring finger) till it touches the root of the thumb. Then press it slightly with the thumb. The third finger, representing water, is stimulated by the electric heat of the thumb representing sun. This posture is useful for person who feel heaviness in the body. It's practice produces imbleness and it should be carried out in both hands while sitting in Padmasana for three or five minutes twice or thrice everyday.[21]

d. ***Jñàna Mudra:***

"The thumb and the index finger are brought together in gentle contact, not necessarily pressing hard against each other. The other fingers are kept upright. This posture must be maintained on both the hands."

"Thjose who suffer form a weak memory, insomnia or a feeling of drowsiness, tension and other maladies of the mind should practice this mudra. It helps to increase mental concentration through constant practice.[22]

Beyond these Mudràs, there are also some other Mudràs mentioned by the Gherand Samhità and by the Hathayoga pradipikà. These Mudràs are not only health giving devices they also awakens the latent universal energy, the Kundallni Sakti. Some of the Mudràs are namely Mahà mudrà, Viparita karani mudra, Nabho mudrà, Khecari mudrà etc. These Mudràs are really very-very difficult to perform but as both of the above mentioned treatises declare they are surely to make physical body free from disease and help in spiritual uplift.

Thus the practice of various mudràs ensures the physical and mental health without introducing any drug into the body.

The healing process of Mantra and Yantra, the integrated parts of Tantra have already been discussed in the previous chapter. These two drugless therapies heal the body-mind complex by strengthening or awakening the inner power of resistance against disease through concentration of mind.

The healing hypothesis which we have made in the Section I, especially, in the Chapter of Tantra sàdhanà, and all these therapies which are based on the concept of Mantra, Yantra and Tantra, more or less based on the Tàntric principle of identical relationship between macrocosm and microcosm. This principle is such a sound and a rational one that by proper manipulation of it, one can escape oneself from the physical, mental and spiritual diseases.

References

1. Translation of the verse taken from the Yoga-Immoratality and Freedom, p. 227 by Eliade, Mircea.

2. Dhauti bastistathà netilaukiki tràkas tatha

Kapalabhàtiscaitàni Satkarmàni samacaret

Gheranda Samhità 1-12. Translated into English by Raibahadur Srisa chandra Vasu, p. 3, 2nd edition, Oriental Book Reprint Corporation, Delhi 1975.

3. Antadhautidantadhauti hridadhauti mùla Sodhanam

Dhauti caturvidhàm krutvà ghatam kurvantu nirmalam

Ibid 1-13.

4. Translation of the verse taken from the Ghernanda Samhità by Rai Bahadur Sirsa Chandra Vasu, pp. 42-43.

5. Abhrakahtava bìjam tu mama bìjam tu pàradah

Ancyobmelanam devi mrutudàridryanàsanam

Resesvara darsanam 6, Sharma, Uma Shankara (Ed.); The Sarva Darsana Samaraba of Madhvàcàrya p. 379. The Vidyabhavan Sanskrit Granthamala 113, Chawkhamba Vidya Bhavan, 1964, First Edition.

6. Sansàrasya param pàram dattessau pàradah smrutah

Ibid, p. 376.

7. Sutosyam matsamoi devi I mama pratyanga sambhavah I

Mama deha raso yasmàt rasatenàmucyate II36II

Rasàrnava Tantra 1-36.

8. Atha vaksyàmi karmàni yoginàm yogasiddhaye

Yànyàha dhùrjatih sàksàllokànugrahahetave II14II

Sat karma samgrah 1.14, Published in the journal of Yoga-Mimàmsà, Vol XI,

No. 1. pp. 1-16, July 1968, Edited and translated by Dr. R. H. Harshe.

9. Ùrdhvacakrì madhyacakrì tathàdhascakrikà parà I

Tràtakam ca kasàkarma netrikaranaamuttamam II15II
Ibid, 1-15.

10. Jalàrdam nijamangustham tàlumadhye pravesayet I
Bharàmayitvà tath pascàttatrastham malamàharet I
Punah punah ksàlaye ccedùrdhva cakrì prakirtità I
Ibid, 1-32-33.

11. Indrago nibham tryasram tàlusthànam ram sucim smaret I
Netrakarnàdyùrdhvarogansanam malasodhanam II34II
Atha vàngulinà kuryàdetat karma mubisvarah I
Ibid, 1-34.

12. Jihvàmùles dhijihvàyàmupajihvàgrata statha II35II
Kanthe càrdràngulim ksiptvà bhràmaye vcàpi pùrvavat I
Malanirharam kurvan pràgvadìrasakham smaran II36II
Madhyacakrì samàkhyàtà kaphakantakanàsinini
Ibid, 1-35-36.

13. Tarjanìm pàyugàm krtvà sodhanam purvavaccaret
Adhascakrì samàkhyàtà yàvadgudavikàssanam I
Yamìram sasakham dhayàtvà sodhayecca yathàvidhi II38II
Mahodaro gulmarogo mùlajà vyàdhayasca ye I
Malàsthathaiva nsayantio bastikarmani yogyata II39II
Ibid, 1-39

14. Sùksmalasye drasu sthàpya nirni mesasciram bhavet I
Asrusampàtaparyantam karma tràtakamìritam I
Vanglàvikaranste sminnantarjyotih prakàsyate I
Netrarogàstathà tandrà nasyantityàha dhùrjatih I
Ibid, 1-40-41.

15. Rajvìn Slaksnàm kasam kuryàddhastamàtràm susùt-rakaih I
Pravesayetkantha madhye nàsadvàrena tàm kasam I
Gharsayecca sanairetatjasàjarma sivoditam I
Anena Karmanà vàyuh kaphadosam harisyati I
Ibid, 1.42-43.

16. Svaccham Slaksnam dradham snigham Svetasùtravinirmitam

Idyà Sampravesyaiva tatah pingalayà haret

Ibid, 1-44.

17. Pràna eva parama mitra pràna eva param sakhà

Prànatulyah parobandhu nàsti nàsti varànane

Siva Svarodaya. Taken from the Sabdakalpadruma.

18. Taken from the article of Acharya Kesha Dev, 'A helping hand for Cardiacs" published in the Times of India, Sunday, October 26, 1980.

19. Ibid.

20. Ibid.

21. Taken from the article of Acharya Kesav Dev, 'The life-giving device", published in the 'Times of India, Sunday August, 1980.

22. Acharya Kesav Dev, 'Your health is in your hands', published in the Times of India, Sunday, February 1, 1981.

CHAPTER - 8

MEANING OF TANTRA

CHAPTER - 8

1. Human Body, A Microcosm

Kosa

The body is supposed to consist of five *kosas* (sheaths), viz, *annamaya* (made of food), *pránamaya* (consisting of vital breath), *manomaya* (made of mind), *vijñánamaya* (consisting of special consciousness), á*nandamaya* (consisting of joy).

Nádis

The body is believed to contain three crores and a half[15] of *nadis* (arteries and veins). Of these, seventy-two are regarded as prominent. Of these again, fourteen or ten are the principal ones. Of these fourteen, the most prominent are *Idá*, *Pingalá* and *Susumná*[16].

The last and the longest one extends from *mñládhára* to *Brahmarandhra* in the head. Also called *brahmanádi*, or *moksamárga*, it is believed to contain the universe. Through it *Kundaliñi* is supposed to move upward. *Idá* is on the left side of the spinal cord. A symbol of the moon, it is white, and represents the *Amrta* aspect of Sakti. Entering *Susumná*, its exit is through the left nostril. *Pingala* is on the right side of the spinal cord. Rising from the *Múládhára*, it ends in the right nostril. Also called *Súrya Nádi*, it symbolises the waking condition, and leads persons to violence.

Cakras[17] — The body is believed to contain six *Cakras* (circle or nerve-plexus). These are as follows:

Múladhára - in the middle of the body, situated in the lowest part of the spinal cord, triangular in shape with its apex downward. It is like a red lotus with four petals. *Kundalini* is supposed to coil around it.

Svádhisthána - above the *múládhára*, but below the navle. It is like a lotus of six patals, presided over by Goddess Rakini.

Manipura - in the navel. It is like a lotus of ten petals, each petal containing a letter. Also called *Nabhicakra*, it contains a triangle of the colour of the rising sun. The outer sides of the triangle are represented by three *Svastika* symbols. It is presided over by a goddess Lakini.

Anáháta - in the region of the heart. It is like a deep red lotus with twelve petals. Seat of air, it is presided over by goddess Kákini.

Visuddha or *Bhárati* - in the region of the neck. Seat of Sarasvati, it is grey and like a lotus of sixteen petals, presided over by goddess Lákini.

Àjñá - between the eyebrows. Also called *Paramakalá* or *Muktatriveni*, it is like a lotus of two petals white in colour. It is from this *cakra* that the three *nádis*, *Idá*, etc., spread out to different directions. Symbolised by the letters *Ha* and *ksa*, it is the seat of mind, presided over by goddess Hakini. The word *Àjña* means order, order of *guru* who is supposed to reside in it.

Cakrabheda or *Satcakrabheda* (literally meaning penetration of *Cakras*) means the manifestation or activation of Cakras; it is necessary for keeping the body fit and for the attainment of *Siddhis*. The six *Cakras* are identified in some Tantric works with the five elements and the mind[18]. This idea appears to have been based on the ancient Upanisadic theories; for example, the heart is compared to a lotus, and it is stated to have 101 *Nadis*; one of them penetrates the crown of the head; a man moving upward by it reaches immortality. In this connexion, the following Upanisads may be consulted; *Chandogya Upanisad*, VIII. I. I, viii.6.6, *Katha* vi.16, Prasna iii.6. Certain diagrams also are called *Cakras*. Different works differ in the names and number of *Cakras*. The *Sricakra* is often mentioned[19]. A Tantra, called *Cakrabheda* (Deccan College MS. No. 962 of 1884-87) mentions the following five *Cakras* used in Durgápájá according to *Kaulágama*.

Rajacakra, Mahácakra, Devacakra, Viracakra, Pasucakra (see *Catalogue*, vol. XVI on Tantra, p. 163). In another manuscript (Deccan College MS. No. 964 of 1887-91) some other *Cakras* are described as *Akadamacakra, Rnadhana, Sodhanacakra, Rasicakra, Naksatracakra*

(*Catalogue*, vol. XVI on Tantra, p. 251).

Sricakra[20], also called *Sriyantra* or *Tripuracakra*, connected with *Srividya*, has been described in verses, quoted in the *Samkara-Vijaya* of Anandagiri (Bib. Indica ed. 1868) p. 255 and in the *Setubandha* commentary on the *Nityásodasikarnava* (1.31-34) quoting from *Yamala* (probably *Rudrayamala*). The *Saundaryalahari* (verse 11) also describes it. A somewhat different description occurs in a work called *Devirahasya* (Deccan College MS. No. 490 of 1895-98). A description of the *Cakra* is as follows. A *Cakra* is to be drawn with the *bindu* in a small triangle. The *bindu* stands for *Sakti* or *Múlaprakrti* solidified. There are nine triangles five of which have their apex downward; these represents *Sakti*, and four, representing *Siva*, have their apex upward. The *bindu* is situated in the smallest triangle pointing downward. There are two pairs of triangles, then 14 triangles, then eight-petalled lotus, 16 petalled lotus, then 3 circles, then three boundary lines with four gates, these ten latter being the outer section of the *Yantra* and the lotuses of 8 and 16 petals being the inner section of the *Yantra*. There is a total of 43 angles. The part of the *Cakra* inside the boundary lines is called *bhupura*. The worship of *Yantra* is *bahiryaga*. *Antaryaga* is taking awakened *Kundalini* through the *Cakras*, from *Muladhara* to *Ájnácakra*, and then uniting it with Siva in the *Sahasrara-cakra*; the six *Cakras* are identified with the five elements and the mind.

Sahasrára Padma[21]

At the centre of the head is located the *Brahmarandhra* through which vital breath or life is supposed to exit at death. It is conceived as a multicoloured lotus of a thousand petals, facing downward.

The *Cakras*, according to the *Kaula* system, are as follows in the ascending order : *Nadicakra* in the *janmasthana*. Based on it is *Máyácakra* in the navel (from here it prevades everywhere), *Yogacakra* (in the heart, centre of yoga), *Bhedanacakra* (in the *tálu* region), *Dipticakra* (*Bindusthána* in between the eye-brows), *Santacakra* (in the nádasthána).

The *Sádhaka* realises it as lustrous like a crore of suns and cool like a crore of moons. By rousing this energy one can reach the higher state of existence. When it is roused, the entire being of a person is flooded with very delicate ambrosia of music; this music is called *Kundalini-kújana* (song of *Kundalini*).

Rele identifies *Kundalini* with the right vagus nerve. But, Woodroffe (Avalon) discards the view; he says that it is not a nerve or any other physical substance or mental faculty; it is rather the ground substance of both. Kuvalayánanda also rejects Rele's theory. The *Rudrayámala* (XXXVI. 6-168) gives 1008 names of *Kundalini*, all beginning with *Ka. Sabdabrahma* is supposed to reside in *Kundalini.*

Besides the individual *Kundalini*, Tantra mentions a *Mahákundali.* The former develops personal existence. By getting upon *Mahakundali* one can transcend the narrow personal state, and establish himself in the wide universal state; *Mahákundali* is at the root of the universe.

2. Human Nautre

In accordance with the preponderance of the qualities of *Sattva*, *Rajas* and *Tamas*, human nature is divided into three classes. On the basis of these qualities, human propensities have been divided into three classes, viz., *Divyabhava*, *Virabhava* and *Pasubhava*.

The *Maitryupanisad* (vi. 21) mentions Susumna Nadi as moving upward. The *Brhádaranyaka* (11.1.19) speaks of 72,000 *Nadis*.

The *Cakras* are sometimes identified with the nerve plexuses of modern physiology. This appears to be wrong in view of the fact that, in Tantra these are imaginary things belonging to the subtle body and not the gross body so that these disappear with the death of a person.

A person, with the preponderance of *Pasubháva*, is tied with the fetters of kindness, infatuation, fear, shame, hatred, family, conduct, caste, etc. In him there is an excess of *Rajas* over *Tamas*. He is forgetful, idle and drowsy. He has no faith in *guru* and *mantra*. He observes Vedic practices. According to Tantra, he is the worst of men. A person, with *Virabháva*, due to the predominance of the quality of *Rajas*, does such acts as lead to grief. One with *Divyabháva*, having the predominance of the quality of *Sattva*, is the best. He is kind, pious, pure, truthful, and has an even attitude towards friends and foes.

3. Sàdhanà—Pañcatattva

Sádhaná (worship, propitiation) is the means to the achievement of *Siddhi* (success, power). The ways of *sádhaná* are *pújá* (external or mental), knowledge of Sástras, *japa* (muttering prayer), *tapas* (penance), *mantra* (incantation), etc.

Sádhakas and *Sádhikás* are divided, in accordance with their physical, mental and moral qualities, into four classes; viz., (1) *Mrdu* (2) *Madhyama* (3) *Adhimatraka* and (4) *Adhimatrama.*

According to the *Kaula* school of Tantra, the *sadhakas* are of the following classes:

1. *Prakrti* — *Virácárin* — engaged in sacrifice and other rituals and resorting to *páncatattvas.*
2. *Madhyama Kaulika* — like Prakrti, with the difference that his mind is more attached to meditation, knowledge and concentration.
3. *Kaulikottama* — those who go beyond ritualism, and meditate on the Supreme Being.

In Tántric worship, *pañcatattva,* also called *Kuladravya* or *Kulatattva,* denoting five *Mararas,* plays an important role. These are *madya*[22] (wine), *mámsa* (meat), *matsya* (fish), *mudrá* (finger-pose), *maithuna* (sexual intercourse).

Some Tantras recommend sexual intercourse when the female partner is in her monthly illness, and her sexual energy is at its peak. For this act, the best place is the funeral ground among the corpses and blazing fire. This is why the female partner is coloured red in representations in art.

As regards the mode of Tántric sexual act, traditions differ,

According to one, perhaps the oldest, the male seed should finally be emitted into the woman's corresponding organ like the offering of scared oil poured into an altar of fire. According to another tradition, the orthodox one, organs must be inhibited, and the energy thus conserved should be turned back and fully sublimated into a radiant inner condition.

The *Sádhaka* of the *Vira* type enjoys these things in their literal sense. Those of the *Pasu* class will take coconut-water or milk, etc., instead of *madya,* red radish, red sesamum, *masúra* (a kind of pulse) in place of fish, ginger, sesamum, salt, or garlic for meat; *mudra,* in this case, denotes barley, rice, etc. Instead of *maithuna,* they will surrender themselves like children to the feet of *Sakti*. For a *Sadhaka* of the *deva* type, *madya*[23] means maddening realisation of the Supreme Being, obtained by *Yoga*, by which he becomes unconscious of the external world. For him, *mámsa* means the action by which he dedicates all arts to himself identified with Brahman.

To him *matsya* means that *Sáttvika* knowledge which enables him to identify himself with all beings, and himself experiences the feelings of pleasure and pain. For him *mudr*á means the giving up of association with all evil things which cause bondage. For such a *sádhaka, maithuna* means the union of the *Kundalinì* energy, residing in *múládhára,*_with the thousand-petalled *Cakra* at the centre of the head.

The *Kulárnava* Tantra gives the following explanation of the *Pañcatattvas; Madya,* called *Tirthávari* in some Tantras, is the nectar flowing from the union of *Kundalinì Sakti* with Siva in the *sahasrara-cakra* in the head[24]. He eats flesh (*mamsa*) who, with the sword of knowledge, kills the animals of merit and demerit, and leads his mind to Supreme Siva. He eats fish who controls his senses, and places them in his Àtman. *Maithuna* means the union of Supreme Sakti and Àtman; Sakti is aroused in a *Kaulika,* but not in a devote of the *pasu* type. *Maithuna* symbolises the basic unity underlying the apparent duality of everything.

The *Mahanirvána* (viii. 170-173) recommends *madhuratraya* (three sweet substances) as substitutes for *madya.* For *Maithuna* it substitutes meditation on the feet of Devi and *japa* of the desired *mantra*.

Pañcatattva is not prescribed for all *Sádhakas*. One, who has reached a highst age of spiritual life, can take a *pañcatattva*, and that also under the guidance of the *guru*. As a safeguard against unrestrained enjoyment of *pancatattvas*, alternative articles are prescribed for those having an excess of animal propensities, and, as such, lacking in the requisite self-restraint. *Pancatattva* is commended for *Sádhakas* of the *Vira* type; they are possessed of self control. Some explain the *makáras* as follows: *Madya* is the stream of nectar issuing from the brain-cavity, the abode of the soul. *Maisya* stands for suppression of vital air.

Mámsa means vow of silence. *Mirthuna* means meditation on creation and destruction.

The *Kaularahasya*[25] appears to describe how the three *Makárás, Madya, Mámsa, Maithuna,* were enjoyed by the common people. It speaks of drinking wine up to throat, eating meat and enjoying beautiful women. Quoting the *Kaularahasya*, the *Hamsavilása* (p. 104) says that *bhoga* and *moksa* do not coexist. But, for one, who enjoys beautiful women, both these come handy.

All, from Bráhmanas to low-class people, are entitled to *Kauladharma* according to the *mahánirvána* (xiv 184).

The *Kaulávali-nirnaya* (V. 113-123) suggests the following substitutes for the *Makáras*. A Bráhmana can use honey in a copper vessel or cow's milk or coconut-water in a bell-metal vessel. In the absence of meat, garlic and ginger can be used. Buffalo-milk or that of the sheep may be used for fish. Roasted fruits and roots may be used for *Maithuna*.

Some[26] are of the opinion that the significance of the *Makáras* was deliberately preverted by vicious people.

It seems that the use of *Makáras* by Tántric devotees brought slur upon Tántric practices. As a result, works like the *Sakti-sangama* started suggesting symbolic interpretations of them.

Tantra recognises the fact that, for progress along the path of

Sádhana, one has to prepare the body, vital breath and mind. The body can be made fit by different postures (á*sanas*). For preparing the vital breath, one has to practice *pránáyáma.* This is prepared by *bhavana* (contemplation).

Three stages of *sádhana* are mentioned. These are

1. *Suddhi*—ridding oneself of physical and mental impurities.
2. *Sthiti*—getting rid of the darkness of delusion and the light of knowledge shining.
3. *Arpana*—realisation of one's identity with the object of meditation.

For a *sádhaka*, essential are *nana, tarpana, sandhy*á, *púj*á and *homa.*

Kundalini-yoga[27]

This is the basic thing for Tántric *sádhana*. The dormant spiritual energy is supposed, to coil round *múládhára* like a serpent[28]. Its gradual ascent, by penetrating the *Cakras*, up to the apex (*brahmarandhra*) is the culmination of *Sádhana.*

Puja

Tantra provides that one must identify oneself with the deity one worships. *Nyása dhyána, japa* are important elements in *púj*á. The offerings may be five to ten in number. In Tantra, *mánasa puja* (mental worship) is regarded as superior to external *puja*. The *Saktananda-tarangini* (vi) says that the search for god outside, having disregarded god within onself is the like the quest of glass ignoring the *Kaustubha* jewel in one's own hand. Self-surrender characteristics Tántric *púj*á.

Siddhi

Siddhi, attainable through *sádhana*, may be of many kinds, e.g., *mantrasiddhi* (Success in *mantras*), *váksiddhi* (success in speech). By the former, *mantra* is made to secure the desired result. By the latter, the speech becomes infallible. After reaching the peak of spiritual life, one can posses the eight *siddhis,* viz., *anim*á (power of assuming an atomic figure), *mahimá* (power of increasing one's size at will), *laghimá* (assuming excessive lightness at will),Isitva (acquiring superority over others), *vasitva* (subduing all to one's will) *Prapti* (obtaining anyting at will) *prakamya* (irresistible will), *kamavasayita* (suppression of passion or desire).

According to the *Mahánirvána* (II. 14-15), Vedic *mantras* led to desired results in *Satya* and other *Yugas*. But, in *Kali* Age, these are like serpents without venom or like dead beings. In this age, Tántric *mantras* yield quick results, and lead to salvation. This Tantra prescribes (iii. 14) that the *mantra Om sac-cid-ekam brahma* in the best; mere perfection in this *mantra* causes the soul to merge in Brahma.

Sometimes, the repetition of a *mantra* is recommended for a lac or even five lac times to ensure great effect like control of even a king.

In some cases, Tantric *mantras* are required to be recited like a Vedic one, with the names of the sage, the meter, the deity and *Viniyoga* (application).

Some Vedic *mantras* also are used in Tantra, but for purposes other than those in the Veda. For example, the mantra *jatavedase sunavama* (Rv. I. 99.1), though addressed to Agni, is employed in invocation to Durgá.

Mantra differs from prayer in that, while the former has fixed syllables, the latter may be said in any form. The syllables of a *mantra* are regarded as the manifestation of Sakti.

Varieties of mantra are called by various names such a *Kavaca, Hrdaya, Astra, Raksá.*, etc.

As seed is sown on a soil which is cultivated and watered, so a *bñja-mantra* is put into a disciple's heart which is pure and has been drenched by the water of God's mercy. The *Mahánirvána* (V. 18-19) states that *Bijas* like *Hrim, Krim* make the form of the deity visible.

Most of the Tantras, particularly the *Parasuráma-kalpasútra Jnánárnava*, the *Sáradátilaka*, hold that *mantras* possess wonderful and incomprehensible power. The *Parasurama-kalpasútra* (1.7.11) mentions faith as the cause of this power. The *Saradatilaka* (II. 57,59) divides *mantras* into three classes, viz., masculine, feminine and neuter. Those ending in *Hum* and *Phat* are male, those ending in *Tha* are female and those ending in *Namas* are neuter.

Purascarana

It literally means performing or carrying out before something. The *Kularnava* (xvii. 87) states that *Purâscarana* is so called because, by the five-fold *upásaná*, the desired deity moves before the worshipper for conferring her favour on him. According to the *Váyaviya-samhitá*, the perfecting of the procedures of the *Múlamantra* is called *Purascarana*, because it has to be performed before the acts in which it is to be employed. In Tantra, it means a rite in which Vedic and Tántric *mantras* are repeated. The *Purascarana* of a *mantra* has the following constituents; *dhyána, pújá, japa, homa, tarpana, abhiseka* and feeding *Bráhmanas.* In a shorter form, the first three are performed. *Dasánga Purascarana* consist in the following additional items: *aghamarsana, suryárghya, jalpana* (*Kaulavalinirnaya* XV). It has been dealt with in many Tantras of which the following are important: *Máhanirvana* (vii. 76.85), Kularava (XV 7-9, 11-12), Sardatilaka (11-138-140) *Ahirbudhnya* (XX.52-53), *Jayakhyasamhitá* (Patala 19, verses 13-33), *Saktisamgama*, Sundari III 155-56, XIV. 45-46, *Gandharva* XXVIII.7-8, *Purascaryárnava*, VI, p. 413, *Kálivilása-tantra* IV,6-7, Krsnanánda's *Tantrasára.*

Raghavabhatta, in his commentary on the *Saradatilaka* (xvi-56), deals exhaustively with details of *Purascarana* that ARE common to all *mantras*.

It is regarded as indispensable for making the *mantra* effective. Raghavabhatta says that as a man, in the grip of a disease, cannot do anything, so a *mantra* without *Purascarana* is abortive.

The places, suitable for this rite, are a holy place, river bank, cave, top of a mountain, confluence of rivers, root of a *Bilva* tree, temple, seashore, any place where one feels happy.

One, performing this rite, is required to eat food obtained by begging (for *Brahmacarin* and *Yati*) *havisyanna*, vegetables, fruits, milk, bulbous roots, barley.

The practices, to be avoided, are sexual intercourse, meat, wine, speaking with women and Sudras.

Japa should be done from morning to noon.

After the rite is commenced, the devotee may encounter obstacles, disturbances and terrible sights. If he remains unmoved, he will achieve miraculous results. If he sticks to the prescribed long time, he will get joy, see pleasant dreams, hear sweet music and enjoy fragrance; these are some of the signs of the perfection of the *mantra*.

There are varying modes of *Purascarana* in accordance with the nature of the devotees, *Pasu, Vira* and *Divya*.

Yoga

In Tantra, *Yoga* is mainly twofold, *hathayoga* and *samádhiyoga*. The former consists in physical discipline paving the way to mind-control.

Hathayoga has the following five accessories instead of the eight prescribed in the *yoga* system of Patañjali.

Yama — control of the senses, non-violence, etc.
Niyama — study of Sástras, meditation on God.
Pránáyáma — control of breath.
Pratyáhára — withdrawl of the sense from the wordly objects.
Asana — a particular posture of the body.
Samádhiyoga is sixfold:
Dhyána, Náda, Rasánanda, Layasiddhi, Bhakti, Rája.

The fundamental difference between the *Yoga* of the *Yogasastra* of Patañjali and *Yoga* in Tantra is this. In Tantra, there is no difference between Sakti and Tattva so that Sakti surmounts all obstacles, and effects the union of the *yogin* with the Supreme Siva. Patañjali, however, does not recognise any Supreme power excepting *Prakrti* so that the *yogin* has no familiarity with any *Sakti* beyond *Prakrti*.

Káya (or Deha) — Siddhi

A fundamental difference between the Bráhmanical Sástra and Tantra is that, while the former ordains physical suffering or self-mortification as a means to the goal, the latter emphasises the value of the body as means to *Sádhaná*. This is not to say that the Bráhmanical Sástra neglects the body. On the contrary, it regards the body as the very first means for the practice of *dharma*. As Kalidasa says (*Kumarasambhava,* V.) *sariram adyam khalu dharmasadhanam.* The *Smrti-sastra* contains elaborate rules for having a good health and recipe for long life. But, it lays a great stress on long fast, arduous and strenuous rites and rituals, abstention from wine, etc., continence and restraint in enjoyments of the objects of sense.

Tantra, however, allows the devotee to indulge in enjoyment of the objects of sense, of course within limits. The core of Tantra *Sadhana* is *mukti* through *bhukti,* a concept absolutely foreign to the orthodox religion and philosophy. Manu unwquivocally states

Pravrttiresá bhútanám nivrttistu maháphalá

There is inclination of creatures for these things; cessatiion of desire, however, leads to great result.

While orthodox Indian philosophy is concerned more with salvation in the other world, Tántric philosophy vigorously advocates *jivanmukti* (liberation in life).

A school of Tántric-Alchemic thinkers used to believe that, by certain yogic processes, *mantras* and chemical drugs, the body of flesh and blood could be made imperishable so that it could defy death. The *Káladahana* and *Mrtyuñjaya* Tantras are stated to contain methods of *Káyasiddhi* (making the body fit or unconscionably longlived).

It is believed that when *káyasiddhi* takes place, the body, strong as *Vajra* and full of youthful lustre, does not become subject to decay, disease and death. The conception is nothing new with the

Buddhists and Alchemists in whose treatises it has been dealt with in detail. The power of *yoga* in rendering the body free from the ills, to which it is ordinarily subjected, has been clearly stated in the following lines of the *Svetásvatara Upanisad* (2, 12);

> *na tasya rogo na jará na mrtyuh*
> *práptasya yogágnimayam sariram*

One, having a body conditioned by *yoga*, has no disease, no decrepitude nor death.

The great efficacy of mercury and mica, in imparting adamantine strength to the body and preserving it for an incredible length of time, has been recognised particularly in the works on alchemy. Mercury is called *Parada*[29] or *Rasa*. It is believed to be Siva's Semen (*Siva-virya*) and mica is supposed to be derived from Sakti.

It is interesting to note that the Natha sect of *Yogins*, traditionally originated by Adinatha and introduced among the people by Matsyendranatha, later influenced by the Bauls and Sahajiya Sadhakas, following the Vajrayana mode, vigorously practised *Kayasiddhi*. The Nathas believed in a process which is briefly this.

The thousand-petalled lotus within the head is turned down. This has to be turned upward by *yoga*. The mind has to be bathed in the nectar contained in that lotus where *Pranava* (*Omkara*) is to be meditated upon. The gateway of *Brahmarandhra* is to be shut. These things being done, the downward flow of ambrosia is checked. This process is called *Akasacandra-bheda* by the *Yogina*. It is supposed that the juice, exuded within the body, is drifted upward by the upblowing wind, and is stored in *Sahasrara*. The believers in this theory admit four kinds of *Candra* (moon), viz., *Adicandra, Nijacandra, Unmadacandra*, and *Garalacandra*. *Nijacandra*, which is of the nature of juice, taken upward, should be united with *Akasacandra* which is attached to *Sahasrara*. Finally, the yogin will drink the *Garalacandra*, which purifies the body and mind, and invigorates the system; this leads to *Siddhadeha*.

The Buddhists and Vaisnava Sahajivas believe in *Kayasiddhi* as the object of *sadhana*.

In the *New Testament* (Book IV); there is mention of supernatural birth, Birth from Above; this is supposed by some to refer to a body obtained by some sort of *kayasadhana.*

FOOT NOTES

1. It is believed that these regions were so named according to the means of transport used in them. *Vishu, Ratha, Asva, Gaja* mean respectively sea-going vessel, chariot, horse and elephant.

For the regions, indicated by these names, see Glossary.

2. Vide *Tantrik Texts*, Vol. 1, ed. A. Avalon, Intro., pp. ii-iv.

3. Vide P. C. Bagchi, *Studies in Tantras*, p. 3, 4.

4. See *Bahvrcopanisad — Saisa para saktih kadividyeti va hadividyeti va sadividyeti.* Also see comm. on it.

5. Vide H. P. Sastri, *Nepal Catalogue*, I. pp. 10, 85, 117.

6. *JASB,* XXVI 1930, pp. 129 f.f.

7. On the question of the priority of Buddhist Tantra over Hindu Tantra or vice versa, see B. Bhattacharya, *Sadhanamala* (Intro., II, P. LXXVIII) and Winternitz HIL II, p. 401.

8. For example, *Harsacrita* (ed. Kane), I. pp. 10, 25, 50 etc., *Kadambari* (ed. Kale), p. 56.

9. Vide Foote, *Collection of Indian Pre-historic and Proto-historic Antiquities,* Madras, 1916; K. R. Subramaniam, *Origin of Savism and its History in Tamil land,* Madras, 1920, Iyenger, *Stone Age in India,* Madras.

10. *HIL*, ii, p. 635.

11. Winternitz, *History of Indian Literature,* I, 1927, p. 591.

12. According to some, the name is the Hinduised form of ka-me-kha, the name of a goddess worshipped by the Khasi tribe in the form of a *yoni* (female organ). See N. N. Bhattacharya, *History of Tantric Religion,* p. 103.

13. Vide *Vanglar Sadhana* by K. M. Sen, pp. 47-48.

14. We shall see that this Tantra originated in Bengal.

15. According to some, 72,000.

16. See *Pranatosini,* I. 4, *Satcakranirupana,* Raghavabhatta's comm. on *Saradatilaka*, xxv. 38.

17. See *Niruttara* X.

18. E.g. *Saundaryalahari,* v. 9

19. See *Sakti* and *Sakta* by Woodroffe (3rd ed.) p. 399, G. Kaviraj describes the system of *Cakras* according to Goraksanatha in *Sarasvatibhavana Studies,* II pp. 83-92. In the translation of *Satcakranirupana* (plates i-vii), Avalon illustrates the six *Cakras* and *Sahasrara* (plate VIII) along with their colours, etc. For Cakras — with illustrations, see C. W. *Leadbeater, Cakras.*

20. See P. V. Kane. *History of Dharmasastra,* V. pt. 2, pp. 1137-38.

21. See *satcakranirupana* XLI-XLIII.

22. Sometimes called *Sura* which, according to *Matrka-bheda-tantra* (iii.40) is so called as it imparts *suratva* (divinity) as soon as drunk.

23. According to some, a preparation of hemp, called *Vijaya* or *Bhang.*

24. This is the view also of the *Kaulajnana-nirnaya* (vi. 18-19) and Bhaskararaya in his comm. on the *Lalitasahasra-nama* (verses 87-91).

25. Deccan College MS. No. 959 of 1884-87 (Copied Samvat 1790-1734 A.D.)

26. E.g. D. N. Bose, *Tantras — their philosophy,* etc., p. 110.

27. For the scientific basis of *Kundalini,* and the attitude of modern scientists to it, see Gop Krishna, *Biological Basis of Religion and Genius,* and its introduction by Weizsacker.

28. It seems to be anticipated by *sarparajni* (serpent-queen) of the *Rgveda.*

29. By Gopinath Kaviraj, reputed as a Tantric *Sadhaka* of a high order. He notes that one, Ramalinga Sastrin of Cidambaram, Madras (Tamil Nadu), who lived about a hundred years ago, attained *Kayasiddhi.* See G. Kaviraj, *Tantric Sadhana O Siddhanta,* II, p. 166.

CHAPTER - 9

THE MYSTERY OF THE NIGHTS

CHAPTER - 9

Sadhana can go on in the dream or sleep state as well as in the waking.

(Sri Aurobindo,-Letters on Yoga, p.1481)

To make use of the nights is an excellent thing, it has a double effect: a negative effect, it prevents you from falling backward, losing whatever you have gained — that indeed, is painful — and a positive effect, you make some progress, you continue your progress.

(The Mother, *Bulletin,* Vol. XII, No.4,p.91)

The Integral Yoga of Sri Aurobindo has for its goal the total transformation of our nature as well as the complete liberation of our being. But in our normal waking state we are conscious only of a very restricted field and action of our nature, the rest of it remaining and functioning behind the opaque veil of our surface personality. But, since all that we 'become and do and bear' in our outer life is prepared and governed by these concealed zones of activity subconscient and subliminal to our waking awareness, it assumes an "immense importance for a yoga which aims at the transformation of life to grow conscious of what goes on within these domains, to be master there and be able to feel, know and deal with the secret forces that determine our destiny and our internal and external growth or decline."

Now, as we have noted before, sleep like yogic trance opens the gate to these subliminal worlds and allows us an entry into the more significant realms of our existence. And although it is a fact that in the ordinary undeveloped state of our consciousness most of our sleep-experience remains unknown to our cognition and even the little that manages to reach our recording surface does so in the form of dreams and dream figures and "not in that condition which might be called an inner waking and which is the most accessible form of the trance state," through a proper and methodical self-disciplining we may grow in consciousness in sleep itself so much so that in the end we may follow in uninterrupted awareness our passage through various realms of our inner being and the return journey therefrom. " At a certain pitch of this inner wakefulness this kind of sleep, *a sleep of experience* can replace the ordinary subconscious slumber."

It is then that we have veridical dreams, dream-experiences of great value, conveying truths that are not so easy to get in our ordinary waking state. Thus problems are solved in our dream consciousness, which our waking consciousness could not possibly cope with; we are provide with warnings and premonitions and indications of the future and with "records of happenings seen or experienced by us on other planes of our own being or of universal being into which we enter."

Our sleep-existence, if we are conscious in it, renders us another valuable service in the exploration of our subconscient nature that contains much that is obscure in us but not distinguishably active in the waking state. A conscious pursuit of the subconscient wanderings of our sleep-consciousness brings to our notice a class of dreams that "arise from the revenge of our inner being freed for a moment from the constraint that we impose on it. These dreams often allow us to perceive some of the tendencies, tastes, impulses and desires of which we would not otherwise be conscious so long as our will to realise our ideal held them down, hidden in some obscure recess of our being." For it is one of the most disconcerting discoveries made in Sadhana that what we have thought to have settled and done away with in the upper layers of our consciousness are obstinately retained by our glutinous subconscient. And just for that reason, as Sri Aurobindo has pointed out, these dreams provide us with a useful indication, for "they enable us to pursue things to their obscure roots in this underworld and excise them."

Hence we see that the fields of our sleep if properly cultivated can yield us a great and effective aid on our road towards self-knowledge and self-mastery, also in the pursuit of our nature-transformation. But how to acquire a cognition of the activities of our nights? How to transform the nature of our sleep?

The procedure to deal with sleep and the dreamland may be said to have three main limbs: (i) how best to enter the state of sleep? (ii) how to remain conscious in sleep itself? and (iii) how to retain the memory of our dream-experiences even when we come back to the waking awareness?

In our quest for the answers to this triple query, to whom else would we turn than to Sri Aurobindo and the Mother, the supreme masters of the fourfold worlds of our being, *jāgrat, svapna, susupti* and *turiya*? So we make no apology for quoting in *extenso* from their luminous writings in an attempt to offer some hints to aspiring seekers.

1. How Best to Enter the State of Sleep?

"You must lie flat on your back and relax all the muscles and nerves....to be like what I call a piece of cloth on the bed, nothing else remains. If you can do that with the mind also, you get rid of all stupid dreams that make you more tired when you get up than when you went to bed. It is the cellular activity of the brain that continues without control, and that tires much. Therefore *a total relaxation,* a kind of *complete calm, without tension* in which everything is stopped. But this is only the beginning.

"Afterwards, a self-giving as total as possible, of all, from top to bottom, from the outside to the inmost, and an eradication also as total as possible of all resistance of the ego, and you begin repeating your mantra — your mantra, if you have one or any other word which has power over you, a word leaping from the heart, spontaneously, like a prayer and that sums up your aspiration. After having repeated a few times, if you are accustomed to it, you *get into trance.* And from that trance you pass into sleep. The trance lasts as long as it should and quite naturally, spontaneously you pass into sleep. But when you come back from this sleep, you remember everything, *the sleep was but a continuation of the trance.*

"Fundamentally the sole purpose of sleep is to enable the body to assimilate the effect of the trance so that the effect may be accepted everywhere, to enable the body to do its natural function of the night and eliminate the toxins. And when it wakes up, there is no trace of heaviness which come from sleep, the effect of the trance continues.

"Even for those who have never been in trance, it is good to repeat a mantra, a word, a prayer before going into steep. But there must be a life in the words, I do not mean an intellectual significa-tion, nothing of that kind, but *a vibration.* And on the body its effect is extraordinary: it begins to vibrate, vibrate, vibrate...and quietly you let yourself go as though you wanted to get into sleep. The body vibrates more and more and still more and away you go."

2. How to Retain the Awareness of Dreams?

The first part of this discipline should naturally deal with the question how to recognise our dreams and, above all, to distinguish between them; for as we have noted before, they vary greatly in their nature and quality. Often in the same night we may have several dreams which belong to different categories and thus have different intrinsic value. Now, as regards the procedure which we should adopt to retain the memory of our nights. Let us listen to the words of the Mother:

"....There is almost always a considerable divergence between what our mental activity actually is and the way in which we per-ceive it, and especially the way in which we remain conscious of it. In its own sphere, this activity determines what vibrations are to be transmitted by repercussion up to the cellular system of our cerebral organ, but in our sleepy brain, the subtle vibrations from the supersensible domain can only affect a very limited number of cells; the inertia of most of the organic supports of cerebral phenomena reduces the number of their active elements, impoverishes the mental synthesis and makes it unfit to reproduce the activity of the internal states other than *by images,* oftenest very vague and inappropriate....

"The cerebral rendering of the activities of the night is at times so much distorted that a form is given to phenomena which is *the exact opposite of the reality...*

"[But] if one knows how to translate in intellectual language the more of less inadequate images by which the brain reproduces these facts, one may learn many things which the too limited physical faculties do not permit us to perceive.

"Some even succeed, by a special culture and training, in acquiring and retaining the consciousness of the deeper activities of their inner being *independently of their cerebral transcription* and are able to recall and know them in the waking state in all the plenitude of their faculties...

"How [then] to cultivate this field of action? how to acquire a *cognition o our activities of the night?...*

"The same *discipline of concentration* which enables a man no longer to remain a stranger to his inner activities in the waking state, also furnishes him with the means of removing the ignorance of those, still richer, of the diverse states of sleep.

"Usually these activities leave only rare and confused memories behind them.

"One finds however that at times a fortuitous circumstance, an impression received, a word pronounced is enough to *reawaken suddenly to consciousness the whole of a long dream* of which the moment before there was no recollection.

"From this simple fact we may infer that our conscious activity participates very feeble in the phenomena of the sleeping state, as in the normal state of things they would remain *lost for ever in subconscient memory...*

"One who wishes to recover the memory of a forgotten dream should in the first place fix his attention on such vague impressions as the dream might have left trailing behind it and follow the indistinct traces as far as possible.

"This regular exercise would let him go farther every day *towards the obscure retreat of the suconscient* where the forgotten phenomena of sleep take refuge and thus ark out a route easy to follow between the two domains of consciousness.

"One practical remark to be made from this point of view is that the absence of memory is very often due to *abruptness* with which the return to consciousness takes place. At this moment, in fact, new activities break into the field of consciousness, drive out forcible all that is foreign to them and afterwards make more difficult the work of concentration necessary to recall the things thus expelled. This is facilitated, on the contrary, whenever certain mental and even physical precautions are observed for a peaceful transition from one state to another."

Thus, the slipping away of the memory of our nights can be greatly remedied and a power developed of going back in memory from dream to dream, from state to state, till a sufficiently coherent knowledge of our sleep life is built up.

But this training of the faculties of memory, as we shall presently see, does not prove sufficient to link the totality of our sleep-existence with our waking awareness. For that we have to grow conscious in the state of sleep itself.

3. How to Grow Conscious in Sleep

The training of our physical memory to follow back the thread of our dream-activities fails to give its full dividend for the simple reason that in this way we are "able to transform into conscious phenomena of the waking state those alone which were already so, be it most fleetingly, during sleep. For *where there was no consciousness, there can be no memory.*

We should therefore seek, in the second place, to extend the participation of consciousness to a greater number of activities in the sleeping state. Now, "the daily habit of going with interest over the various dreams of the night, this transforming their vestiges little by little into precise memories as well as that of noting them down on waking are very helpful from this point of view.

"By virtue of these habits, the mental faculties will be induced to adapt their mechanism to the phenomena of this order and to direct upon them their attention, curiosity and power of analysis.

"It will then produce a sort of *intellectualisation of dream,* achieving the double result of interspersing the conscious activities more and more intimately in the play, hitherto disordered, of the activities of the sleeping state and of augmenting progressively the scope of these activities by making them more and more rational and instructive.

"Dreams would then take on the character of precise visions and, at times, of dream revelations."

But along with this participation of mental consciousness, this revelatory intellectualisation of dreams, we must try to cultivate a still higher and deeper mode of consciousness in sleep. In fact, our sleep-life should be as much a part of Sadhana as the waking one, and the developing consciousness that we attain in our waking state through spiritual endeavor and aspiration should extend itself fully and continuously also to the sleep state. It is true that at the beginning and for a long time it becomes difficult to maintain the consciousness at the same pitch at night, for "the true consciousness comes at first in the waking state or in meditation, it takes possession of the mental, the vital, the conscious physical, but the subconscious vital and physical remain obscure and this obscurity comes up when there is sleep or an inert relaxation." But with the growth of an intense Sadhana in our waking state, when we develop our inner being, live from in without and our subconscient is enlightened and penetrated by the Mother's light, this disparity and this dislocation of consciousness disappears, and our "sadhana goes on in the dream or sleep state as well as in the waking."

4. The Lure of the Dream-Consciousness

At this point of our discussion we would like to address a note of warning to the seekers after the mastery of their nights.

Through a proper cultivation of the fields of sleep-existence, when the inner sleep consciousness begins to develop and along with it appear dream experiences as distinct from ordinary dreams, there is often an irresistible pull on the consciousness to withdraw from its waking status, go within and follow the development there even when there is no fatigue or need of sleep — so alluring are the experiences of dream-consciousness, so overwhelming is the charm thereof!

But this attraction of the sleep-world must not be allowed to encroach on the waking hours and the "wanting to get back to something interesting and enthralling which accompanies the desire to fall into sleep" should be effectively curbed. Otherwise there may be an undesirable unbalancing and "a decrease of the hold on outer realities."

CHAPTER - 10

The Vision of the Divine Body

CHAPTER - 10

The Light now distant shall grow native here,
The Strenght that visits us our comrade power;
The Ineffable shall find a secret voice,
The Imperishable burn through Matter's screen
Making this mortal body godhead's robe

(Sri Aurobindo, *Savitri,*Book II, Canto II,p.110)

Past and gone are three mortal generations: the fourth and last into the Sun will enter.

*(Rig-Veda,*VIII. 102. 14)

If the transformation of the body is complete, that means no subjection to death — it does not mean that one will be bound to keep the same body for all time. One creates a new body for oneself when one wants to change...

(Sri Aurobindo, *Letters on Yoga*,p.11)

The Integral Yoga of Self-Transformation as revealed to man by Sri Aurobindo and the Mother has for its aim, in contradistinction to the attempts mentioned in the foregoing chapter, the creation of a divine body, here in the conditions of earth and matter. It does not want to be contented with a cinmayadeha,or transcendental body, as in the case of the Vaishnavas, nor with the possession of a post-mortem 'pneumatic' body of Pauline conception.

For, this Yoga aims not at a release from embodied existence (as even the Tantra and Vaishnavism do at the end), at a departure out of the world into some supraterrestrial world of bliss and spiritual enjoyment, but at a change of earthly life and existence, at a divine fulfilment of life here upon earth, and that, and that too "not as something subordinate of incidenta[l], but as a distinct and central object". Also, "the object sought after [in this Yoga] is not an individual achievement of divine realisation for the sake of the individual, but something to be gained for the earth-consciousness here."

Now, in this framework of the goal of a divine fulfilment of terrestrial life, the importance of the body is indeed obvious. For, as Sri Aurobindo himself has decared:

"A total perfection is the ultimate aim which we set before us, for our ideal is the Divine Life which we wish to create here, the life of the Spirit fulfilled on earth, life accomplishing its own spiritual transformation even here on earth in the conditions of the material universe. That cannot be unless the body too undergoes a transformation, unless its action and functioning attain to a supreme capacity" and "the physical consciousness, and physical being, the itself...be suffused with a light and beauty and bliss from the Beyond and the life divine assume a body divine."

Elsewhere Sri Aurobindo sounds a note of warning: "It is because he has developed of been given a body and brain capable of receiving and serving a progressive mental illumuination that man has risen above the animal. Equally, it can only be by developing a body or at least a functioning of the physical instrument capable of receiving and serving a still higher illumination that he will rise above himself and realise, not merely in thought and in his internal being but in life, a perfectly divine manhood. Otherwise either the promise of Life is cancelled, its meaning annulled and earthly being can only realise Sachchidananda by abolishing itself, by shedding from it mind, life and body and returning to the pure Infinite, of else man is not the divine instrument, there is a destined limit to the consciously progressive power which distinguishes him from all other terrestrial existences and as he has replaced them in the front of things, so another must eventually replace him and assume his heritage."

But fortunately for earth-life and for man neither of these altenatives need be envisaged. For man has convincingly shown by his past achievement that he is capable in all parts of his being of exceeding *ad infinitum* the bounds of his actuality. Thus there is no inevitability of logic why he himself should not at the glorious prospect of divine manhood, by opering all his members, — his mentality, his life, and, the last but not the least, his body itself, — to the unveiled action of the Supermind and allowing them to be integrally moulded and transfigured by that 'greater term of the Spirit manifesting in Nature.'

For, it should be clearly borne in mind that the divine body thus envisaged can come into existence and its physical immortality be achieved and assured, not through the paltry efforts made by science, nor through the occult-spiritual influences that seek to act upon Mtter through the sole agency of the powers of consciousness so far organised in earth-nature, but through the action of the Supramental Power, the power of "the fall Truth-Consciousness of the Divine Nature". This Truth-Consciousness, *rta-cit,* the Supermin as Sri Aurobindo terms it, is "a dynamic and not only a static Power, not only a Knowledge, but a Will according to Knowledge," that can "manifest direct its world of Light and Truth in which all is luminously based on the harmony and unity of the One, not disturbed by a veil of Ignorance".

Also, when this Supramental Power overtly intervenes in the field of body and Matter, its working will be "not an influence on the physical giving it abnormal faculties, but an entrance and penetration changing it wholly into a supramentalised physical".

Now, as regards the nature and character of this supramentalised physical making possible the appearance, here upon earth itself, of a wholly transfigured divine body, Sri Aurobindo has written in great detail in the penultimate chapter of *The Life Divine* and, more exhaustively, in his last work *The Supramental Manifestation upon Earth.*

The limited span of the present work does not permit us to discuss in full the nature of this apotheosis of the material body of man, as envisaged in the Yoga-Philosophy of Sri Aurobindo and the Mother, nor can we indicate how for and in what way the insistent problems of food and sleep, fatigue and inertia, disease and decay, unregenerated impulses and appetites are going to be solved in the transformed divine body to appear in time. We content ourselves with picking up here one theme, *the* theme, we might as well say, of the Sphinx-like problem of death sn dissolution of the individual's physical body.

For, we have been assured by Sri Aurobindo and the Mother that as a crowning achievement of the Supramental Manifestotion upon Earth, there will come will come about 'the physical conquest of death, an earthly immortality',—"in the sense not of attachment or of restriction to our present corporeal frame but an exceeding of the law of the physical body." For, "from the divine Bliss, the original Delight of existence,the Lord of Immortality comes pouring the wine of that Bliss, the mystic Soma, into there jars of mentalised living matter; eternal and beautiful, he enters into these sheaths of substance for the integral transformation of the being and nature".

And thus will be realised for man his age-old yearning, "the consummation of a triple immortality,—immortality of the nature completing the essential immortality of the Spirit and the psychic survival of death,"—which will be "the crown of rebirth and a momentous indication of the conquest of the material inconscience and Ignorance even in the very foundation of the reign of Matter,... a temporal sign of the spirit's victory here over Death and Matter".

But before this vision of the conquest of Death, can be realised in the life of man, the metaphysical necessity for its existence and away so far has to be adequately met and abrogated.

So our task now is to proceed to the study of the metaphysics of death and indicate the condition necessary for the attainment of a physical immortality.

CHAPTER - 11

THE CONQUEST OF SLEEP

CHAPTER - 11

Thine is the shade in which visions are made;
sped by thy hands from celestial lands
come the souls that rejoice for ever.
Into thy dream-worlds we pass or look in thy magic glass,
then beyond thee we climb out of Space and Tıme
to the peak of divine endeavour.

(Sri Aurobindo, *Collected Poems and Plays,* Vol. II,p.122)

He has seen God's slumber shape these magic worlds.
He has watched the dumb God fashioning Matter's frame,
Dreaming the dreams of its unknowing sleep,
And watched the unconscious Force that built the stars.
He has learnt the Inconscient's workings and its law...
Its somnolence founded the universe,
Its obscure waking makes the world seem vain...
He must call light into its dsrk abysms,
Else never can Truth conquer Matter's sleep
And all earth look into the eyes of God.

(Sri Aurobindo, *Savitri,* Book VI, Canto II, pp. 449-50)

We have seen in the course of our study of *longue haleine* on the occult nature and function of sleep that the periodic spells of dormancy of our body *need not* prove to be an unavoidable evil nor a handicap to our spiritual growth. In any case, our physical sleep does not *necessarily* mean an abeyance of consciousness of the whole of our dynamic being, nor a nightly falling down, nor even an interruption in the pursuit of our Sadhana. On the other hand, this may be transformed, if we know how to do it, into a *sleep of experiences* giving us an access to the inner domains of our being.

But whatever may be the value of the sleep-existence, to live in the dream-world at the price of the suspension of our waking awareness cannot be considered a laudable achievement in the Yoga of Transformation of Life. We have to bring out and call down the reaches from our subliminal depths and superconscient height and make these an acquisition of our waking life. Our physical consciousness has to be "spiriturally awake" and "as open in thc waking consciousness as in sleep." We have some how to "arrive at a point when one remains outwardly conscious and yet lives in the inner being and has at will the indrawn or the outpoured condition."

It is thus evident that the irresistible bouts of unconsciousness of sleep to which our body's waking status occasionally succumbs cannot but be viewed as a sign of imperfection in the prevailing organisation of our physical being. What is then necessary is that — and this must constitute an essential element in the total transfiguration of our bodily existence — *sleep mist be raised from the level of necessity to that of a free acceptance,* as and when so willed, as an indrawn absorption of our consciousness.

Thus the mastery over our nights should be followed by the attempt at an absolute conquest of sleep. But is this total victory over physical sleep at all feasible in the present human body? And, if not, what are the essential conditions that have to be met before this prospect for bodily life enters the field of realisable possibilities?

By way of answering these crucial questions we propose to put forward two related problems and venture some tentative solutions thereof.

1. How to Reduce the Hours of Sleep?

On the purely physical-vital plane, sleep has for its essential function the restoration of the nervous physical energies of our fatigued bodily system. But for an effective fulfilment of this function, it is absolutely necessary that our sleep-life should be calm and reposeful, relaxed and luminous. But very rarely do our nights measure up to this criterion: these are, more often than not, more fatiguing than even our days for reasons which often escape us.

But the Mother has warned us that if we get up not so well refreshed in the morning, it is because of a formidable mass of Tamas. "It is Tamas which causes bad sleep. There are two kinds of bad sleep: the sleep that makes you heave, dull, as though you lose all the effect of the effort you put in during the preceding day; and the sleep that exhausts you as if you were passing your time in fight.

"...Two things you must eliminate: falling into the torpor of the inconscience, with all these things of the subconscient and of the inconscient that rise up, invade you, enter into you; and a vital and mental superactivity where you pass your time in fighting literally terrible battles. People come out of that state bruised, as if they had received blows — and they did receive them, it is not 'as if'!"

(A) Relaxation: Now, since the total time interval needed for the recuperation of our energies is in inverse ratio to the quality of repose that we attain in our sleep, the very first procedure we must adopt to cut down the duration of our nightly sleep is to practise the art of complete relaxation of body and mind, a short period of which proving to be more refreshing than hours of restless sleep. In the recommendation of a Buddhist author: "Relax each portion of the body deliberately and consciously; then close the eyes and try to visualise utter darkness. Feel yourself floating in a silent void, and deliberately empty the mind of every thought and feeling by imagining such a condition as Swinburnes's "Only a sleep eternal in an eternal night." And the author concludes that, once the proper knack is abundance of fresh energy and a clean-swept invigorated mind.

Be that as it may, this negative method of relaxation cannot take us very far on our road to the conquest of sleep. It should from rather the essential preliminary step to a for more effective and spiritually beneficial one: to become conscious in our sleep and deliberately utilise our nights for progress.

(B) Conscious utilisation of nights: At this point we would like to dispel a possible misunderstanding that may arise in connection with this suggestion for a conscious utilisation of our nights. There may be a lurking fear in some minds that this attempt at the cultivation of the vast fields of our nights, instead of bringing in a more reposeful and therefore a more invigorating, sleep would on the other hand affect its depth and detract from the efficacity of our nightly rest which is so salutary and indispensable for our physical

health.

But this fear and doubt have got no basis in fact. For, as the Mother has assured us, it is only the useless and uncontrollable and mostly subconscious activities in our sleep that make our nights more fatiguing than the day. On the contrary, "if our night granted us the acquisition of new knowledge, the solution of an absorbing problem, the establishment of contact in our inner being with some centre of life or of light, or even the accomplishment of some useful work, we should always get up with a feeling of vigour and well-being. It is the *hours wasted in doing nothing useful of good that are the most fatiguing.*"

This conscious cultivation of our sleep-existence for reaping fruits for our inner growth is then the second essential element of our endeavour to make the state of physical sleep a real restorer of our energies.

But the gain acquired even in this way seems to be limited in its scope so far as our main problem of drastically reducing the hours of sleep is concerned. For that we have to become conscious masters of another significant phenomenon of our sleep-life: the possibility of entrance into the "*susupti* of Brahman of Brahmaloka."

(C) Attainment of Sachchidananda immobility: Once before we have already made a passing reference to this state of luminous rest in sleep. As a matter of fact, for sleep to be at all worth the name fulfilling its role of the restorer of energies, it must be either one "in which there is a luminous silence" or else one "in which there is Ananda in the cells." The rest of our sleep-life is an *attempt at sleep, not sleep* itself. To quote from the Mother a passage to which we have already referred:

"There is the possibility of a sleep in which you enter into an absolute silence, immobility and peace in all parts of your being and your consciousness merges into Sachchidananda. You can hardly call it sleep for it is extremely conscious. In that condition you may remain for a few minutes, but these *few minutes give you more rest and refreshment than hours of ordinary sleep.*"

Sri Aurobindo too has treated this topic on numerous occasions. Thus, to quote from him only one passage:

"In sleep one...passes from consciousness to deeper consciousness in a long succession until one reaches the psychic and rests there of else from higher to higher consciousness until one reaches rest in some silence and peace. *The few minutes one passes in this rest are the real sleep* which restores, — if one does not get it, there is only a half rest."

But, as a matter of fact, this brief Sachchidananda period of "luminous and peaceful dreamless rest" that "gives sleep all its restorative value" cannot be had "by chance; it requires a long training." Indeed, our ordinary sleep, even when it is of the best variety, is mostly taken up with our actual *travelling* towards this state of Sachchidananda immobility and our return journey to the waking awareness, without very often ever reaching the state at all.

And even if we reach this state on some rare occasions, "it is done unconsciously as it is. If one wants to do it consciously and regulate it, one has first to become conscious in sleep." And then alone can the prospect possibly open up before us of reducing the hours of sleep to a bare minimum.

But even this cannot altogether eliminate the necessity of sleep. The reason is twofold, physiological and occult-spiritual, to whose consideration we now turn.

2. How to Eliminate the Necessity of Sleep?

Physical precondition: On the purely physico-physiological plane, since sleep is the body's unavoidable response to its overstrain and exhaustion through an ill-balanced expenditure of energy, what is needed is the total annulment of all possibility of our body's fatigue. And this brings us to the general problem of incapacity and inertia of our present physical organisation. For, although it is a fact that "either the yogic or the vital energy can long keep at work an overstrained or declining physical system, a time comes when this drawing is no longer so easy nor perhaps possible" and the bad results long held back from manifesting explode all at once and a breakdown ensues.

So the problem of incapacity has to be tackled and soved on the plane of the body itself. For "the body is the key, the body the secret both of bondage and of release, of animal weakness and of divine power, of the obscuration of the mind and soul and of their illumination, of subjection to pain and limitation and of selfmastery, of death and of immortality."

But what is the inherent reason for this fatigue of our body? Why does our physical system get periodically tired? Why can it not work in a continuous way?

In the words of the Mother:" The fatigue of the body comes from an inner disharmony. There may be many other *apparent reasons,* but all amount to that fundamental circumstance."

What is this want of harmony due to? The answer lies in the fact of a limited life-force, lodged in the confines of a limited and egobound individualised existence, contending in vain with the universal All-Life and All-Force that seeks constantly to govern and master it. In the evolutionary emergence and development of life in material forms, it is true that as consciousness develops more and more, "as the light of its own being emerges from the enert darkness of the involutionary sleep, the individual existence becomes dimly aware of the power in it and seeks ferst nervously and then mentally to master, use and enjoy the play."[4] But, even at our best, we mental beings are bound are bound by a poor and limited life power which is all that our body can bear or to which it can give scope. And" in the consequent interchange and balancing between the movement and interaction of the vital energies normally at work in the body and their interchange with those which act upon it from outside, whether the energies of others or the general Pranic force variously active in the environment, there is a constant precarious balancing and adjustment which may at any moment go wrong."[5]

Thus, in the very nature of things, our individualised life and force in the body cannot master the All-Force working in the world.

On the contrary, the resistance which it offers through blind ignorance to the movement of the infinite universal Life "with whose total will and trend its own will and trend may not immediately agree",[1] subjects it to the law of incapacity and fatigue, one of the basic characteristics of individualised and divided Life in the body.

Hence to cure our physical system of all liability to fatigue, the limitation of ego has to be totally abrogated not only in the inner parts of our being, but in the very physical consciousness and the material organisation of the body. Our body has to be brought into complete harmony with the demands of our own inner consciousness and with the infinite cosmic rhythm.

But "that means", in the words of the Mother, " a work in each cell of the body, in each small activity, in each movement of the organs... You have to enter into the disposition of the cells, your inner physical organisation if the body is to answer to the Force that descend.. You must be conscious of your physical cells, you must know their different functions, the degrees of receptivity in each, which of them are in good condition and which are not."

But this cannot be attempted with the help of the insufficient and inefficient light of mind-consciousness. It is only through the descend and concomitant emergence of the divine Gnosis, Supermind, here in the midst of the evolutionary Becoming, that Matter and material body can be rid of their inertia and inconscience and a proper equation established between he life-energy playing in an individual formation and the surges of the embarking All-Force. For in the Supermind "alone is the conscious unity of all diversities; there alone will and knowledge are equal and in perfect harmony; there alone Consciousness and Force arrive at their divine equation."

It is through the supramental transformation of our physical body,—that "is still a flower of the material Inconscience."[4]— down to its very cells and functioning that the law of incapacity and consequent fatigue will be finally abrogated and with it the physiological compulsion for sleep.

But there remains a final hurdle, the occult-spiritual necessity of sleep, but that too will be completely annulled with the gnostic transformation of our waking existence.

Occult-spiritual precondition: We have seen that in its essential nature our body's sleep is the response to the demand of the individual consciousness to go inward and awake in planes of existence not at present accessible to the waking awareness which is still in the grip of an involutionary half-sleep. So, unless and until his spiritual slumber is totally eliminated from all parts of the being including our very physical consciousness, mother Nature will constrainour body to fall occasionally into the swoon of slumber so that the portals of the inner and higher life can open.

Now, when Supermind or Gnosis, the Truth-Consciousness of Sachchidananda, overtly emerges in the field of evolution to become the governing principle of our embodied material existence, the manifested being will be in secure possession of an integral Consciousness and an integral Sight, so that there will be no more a state of sleep in opposition to the state of permanent waking, nor for that matter a line of demarcation separating the inner and outer domains of existence. The evolving being will then be fully aroused from the self-oblivion of an involutionary sleep and, along with it, the spiritual compulsion behind the sleep of our body will altogether lose its occult support.

In that foresble Golden Dawn, the body will thrill with the fulfilment of its destiny, it will participate in full awareness in the glories of a divinised life upon earth and the law of the inexorable necessity of sleep will be for ever lifted from its head.

But in the meantime let us not forget even for a moment the great role that sleep can play in the present organisation of our life and being; for, does it not open to us the doors of the dream-land, the Yogic dream-world, if we only know how to put it to service?

And who can be little the infinite charm and beauty and bliss that the Mother of Dreams may bestow upon us, if we only know how to court Her favour?

APPENDIX

THE MOTHER OF DREAMS*

SRI AUROBINDO

Goddess supreme, Mother of Dream, by the ivory doors when
thou standest,
Who are they then that come down unto men in thy visions that
troop, group upon group, down thc path of thc shadows slant-
ing?
Dream after dream, they flash and they gleam with the flame of
the stars still around them;
Shadows at the side in a darkness ride where the wild fires
dance,
stars glow and glance and the radom meteor glistens;
there are voies hat cry to their kin who reply; voices sweet,
at heart they beat and ravish the soul as it listens.
What then are these lands and these golden sands and these
seas
more radiant than earth can imagine?
Who are those that pace by the purple waves that race to the
cliff-bound floor of thy jasper shore under skies in which
mystery muses,
Lapped in moonlight not of our night or plunged in sun shine
that
is not diurnal?
Who are they coming they Oceans roaming with sails whose
strands
are not made by hands, an unearthly wind advances?
Why do they join in a mystic line with those on the sands
linking
hands in strange and stately dances?
Thou in the air, with a flame in thy hair, the whirl of thy won-
ders
watching,
Holdest the night in thy ancient right, Mother divine,
hyacinthine,

with a girdle of beauty defended.
Sworded with fire, attracting desire, thy tine bours kingdom thou keepest,
Starry-sweet, with the moon at thy feet, now hidden now seen the clouds between the gloom and the drift of thy tresses.
Only to those whom thy fancy chose, O thou heart-free is it given to see thy wetch craft and fell they caresses.
Open the gate where thy children wait in their world of a beauty undarkened.

High-throned on a cloud, victorious, proud I have espied
Maghavan ride when the armies of wind are behind him;

Food has been given for my tasting from heaven and fruit of immortal sweetness;

I have drunk wine of the kingdoms divine and have heard the change of music strange from a lyre which our hands cannot master;

Doors have swung wide in the chambers of pride where the

Gods reside and the Apsaras dance in their circles faster and faster.

For thou art she whom we first can see when we pass the bounds of the mortal,

There at the gates of the heavenly states thou hast planted thy wand enchanted over the head of the Yogin waving.

From thee are the dream and the shadows that seem and the fugitive lights that delude us;

Thine is the shade in which visions are made; sped by thy hands from celestial lands come the souls that rejoice for ever.

Into thy dream-worlds we pass or look in thy magic glass, then beyond thee we climb out of Space and Time to the peak of divine endeavour.

CHAPTER - 12

ATTEMPTS AT 'KAYASIDDHI' AND REJUVENATION

CHAPTER - 12

Then man was born among the monstrous stars
Dowered with a mind and heart to conquer thee.

(Sri Aurobindo, *Savitri,* Book IX, Canto II, p. 594)

The Ars magna, *that royal and sacerdotal science of the alchemists, is verily a science of regeneration... Many a seeker on the ways of the Divine has undergone spiritual regeneration. But very few are they who have known the mystery of corporal renewal.*

(D.Eckhartshausen, La Nuee sure Le Sanctuaire)

Senescence and natural death, '*la mort naturelle*', are thus seen to be not at all necessary and intrinsic attributes or accompaniments of incarnate life. Hence have arisen on the part of man various deliberately planned attempts at the physical and practised in the modern West, — this battle for the victory over senile decay and the body's death is no longer considered to be farcical and futile, but rather as a veritable scientific problem and proposition. Already in the year 1924, S. Metalnikov of the Institute Pasteur (Paris) wrote: "All efforts of the biologist and medical men to wage a successful battle against the onset of senescence and restore youth to the aged and decadent ought to be considered as practically possible and scientifically motivated *(prejudgement possibles et scientifiquement motivees)*"

Here we may briefly state them a in attempts, both scientific and occult-spiritual, that have been so far made for the physical conquest of death.

(A) *Rejuvenation Procedures:* Indeed, in recent years, science has proceeded in right earnest to tackle the problem of aging and death, starting from the lower end of the range of our being.

It has sought to formulate theories, and act effectively, on the underlying physico-chemical factors and processes that govern the phenomenon of progressive senescence of the body-locked soma-cells and have for their ultimate and inexorable consequence the somatic death of the individual organism. In our time much valuable work has been ne in this specialized field of biology and the interested reader may consult appropriate publications for relevant information.

In brief, we may state that many are the theories that have been put forward to explain the onset of the phenomenon of senescence (e.g., those of Maupas, Hertwig, Mainot, Koltzoff, Metchnikof, Weissmann and others), and numerous have been the attempts to achieve rejuvenation of the aging body and lengthen the span of life[1] by various surgical alterations of certained endocrinal organs, particularly the essential organs of sex.

Indeed, it has often been thought that aging is brought about by the failure of one or other of the endocrine glans and attempts have been made to rejuvenate an aging body by grafting to it appropriate glands or injecting into it glandular extracts.

But, from the fundamental point of view, these have by no means solved the problem at its base. For, on the one hand, no theory of sineil decline so far put forward can be regarded as entirely satisfactory or as generally established by the evidence. Also, "most of them suffer from the logocial defect of setting up some particular observed attribute or element of the phenomenon of senescence itself, such as protoplasmic hysteresis, slowing rate of metabolism (meaning essentially only reduced activity), etc as the cause of the whole".

One the other hand, whatever may have been the immediate physical and psychological effects of the procedures of rejunvenation, these have proved to be no more than temporary heightening of some gland activities, altogether "transient results" as one distinguished biologist has termed them. There is as yet no evidence whatsoever that these medico-scientific procedures help to increase in any way the basic potential specific longevity of the individual. In the words of Prof. Vernon T. Schuhardt, an authority in the field:

"Although loudly proclaimed, these procedures were not well founded in theory and have not with stood the exacting the critical tests of time and confirmation. No evidence has been discovered that a the aging the body *as a whole* is dependent on either the activity or the failure o the sexual glands, *per se* . . . The effects were temporary and did not offset the slow decline of old age. Indeed, some danger is involved in such a one-sided stimulation of the senile since the organism as a whole may not be physically constituted to withstand the sudden and abnormal stress... The hormones may alter the background of physiological reactions and modify that structural integrity of the cells and tissue, but they have *little lasting effect on the primary causes of aging the senility...* Thus while the germinal elements become the source of posterity, the body seems predestined to weaken, grow old and die. And by the latter 1950's nomeans have been found to seriously alter this decline."

So we see that the scientific attempts at preventing devitalisation and prolonging the individual life-span of man have so far proved futile and illusive, and we on our part venture to assert that these will prove equally so even in the future; for, the root of the malady lies somewhere else and is too deep and inscrutable for science to probe or to find the remedy thereof. To anticipate the line of suggested solution, we may state forthwith that "even if Science -physcial Science or occult Science—were to discover the necessary conditions or means for an indefinite survival of the body, still, if the body could not adapt itself so as to become a fit instrument of expression for the inner growth, the soul would find some way to abandon it and pass on to a new incarnation. *The material or physical* causes of death are not its sole or its true cause; its true inmost reason is the spiritual necessity for the evolution of a new being."

(B) *Kāyāsiddhi procedures:* Leaving behind the field of scientific achievements as well as failures,we pass onnow to a surrmary consideration of some of the attempts made by man, starting from the other, the higher, end of the range of our being.

These occult-spiritual attempts at *dehasiddhi,* the attainment of perfection of the material body of man, have in the majority of cases come down to us in the form of traditions and a lore whose sources sometimes have been lost in the obscure and remote past of the race.

Thus, in the words of the Mother, "in a very ancient tradition, preceding even the Vedi and Chaldean traditions, there was already the question of a glorious body which would be plastic enough to be constantly remodelled by the deeper consciousness, a body expressing this consciousness. There was the question of luminosity: the matter constituting the body being able to become luminous at will. There was the question of a kind of lightness being possible which would enable the body to move about in the air by mere will-force and some procedure of handling the inner energy on so on."

Some Buddhist traditions speak of the Buddha's temporary victory over death, *Mrtyumãra.* These are based on a Buddhist belief that ust as an *arhat* can abandon the 'coefficients of life,' so he can also stop them (*sthãpayati*). "According to the Vaibhasikas, the saint says: 'May [the action that is to ripen for me in enjoyment ripening life!' By its nature, life is 'ripening' (*vipãka),* and it can replace any enjoyment which normally ought to ripen from a former merit, and which the saint no longer desires and has escaped by his sainthood. By this process, 'vanquishing death', the Buddha prolonged his life three months for the salvation of men, and the disciples employ this to assure the duration of the *dhamma* . This term of three months seems to be given as a maximum, ad as the mark of the victory of the Buddha over *Mrtyumãra,* 'Mara, who is death'."[1]

This question of a possible maximum limit to the postponement of death is very significant and highly germane to the problem we have been discussing. For, although there have been in the past "seemingly allied ideas and anticipation—the perfectibility of the race, certain Tantric sadhanas, the fort after a complete physical siddhi by certain schools of yoga, " these have been attempted for the most part as indiviudal personal achievements, imperfect and precariously maintained by the help of Yogasiddhis, and not as a *dharma,* natural law, of the transformed physcial nature. But "mental or vital occult power", warns Sri Aurobindo, "can only bring siddhis of the higher plane into the indiviudal life— like the Sannyasi who could take any poison without harm, but he *died of a* poison after all when he forgot too observe the conditions of the siddhi."

Among the various attempts in the past falling into this category, mention may be made of:

(i) attempts at *dehasiddhi* through *kãlabañcana,* conquest of Time, by certain schools of Hathayoga;

(ii) attempts at the attainment of a *rasamayi tanu,* body with divinessence, by the Raseswara sect;

(iii) attempts at skandasiddhi made by certian Mahayani Tantric schools among the Buddhists;

(iv) attempts at *kãyãsiddhi* by Nathayogis like Matsyendra, Goraksha, Jalandharanath and others;

(v) attempts at the elaboration of a *bhãvadeha* by Sahajiya Vaishnavas.

But none of these attempted Siddhis became intrinsic to the material body and hence cold not be made to endure. As a matter of fact, as we shall see in the course of our study, "there can be no immortality of the body without supramentalisation; the potentiality is there in the yogic force and yogis can live for 200 or 300 years or more, but there can be no real principle of its without the supramental."

CHAPTER - 13

Rare Siddhis

CHAPTER - 13

1. Ashtottarshat Naamaani

The musk deer keeps roaming here & there throughout ..... it does feel a fragrance but never succeeds in finding its source. The mankind too can smell a wonderful fragrance... Only if it could know that its source is present between its very midst.

India has been holding the torch of the spiritual leadership of the world since ages and the ancient Indian science & knowledge has always enlightened the path of spiritualism. No other nation has such a glorious and rich heritage and no other culture has affected the minds of those seeking peace & enlightenment so much, as has been done by the Indian culture. The reason for this has been the deep knowledge & philosophy possessed by the sages and ascetics of India, through which they attained several Siddhis or spiritual accomplishments and also acquired such powers through Sadhanas, so as to bless anyone with a happy and contented life. These great men were able to control all the powers in the nature through penance and proved by achieving totality of life that one can maintain a harmony between spirituality and materialism in one's life.

Due to the changing times and the onslaught of foreign culture there occurred depreciation in the traditional values and even the moral & human values. As a result the spirituality prevalent in the society became extinct, but even after so much degradation these knowledges did not vanish altogether. Even today, a great ascetic, a great philosopher, a great scholar and an exponent of those traditions is present amidst us. And this great personality does not just have a superficial knowledge of these ancient Indian sciences but has a deep & firm grasp on them.

There are several knowledges and Siddhis which have brought so much fame & respect to the Indian culture and nine of these are considered to be main.

2. Parkaya Pravesh

Parkaya Pravesh means entering one's soul in the body of some other person. Through this knowledge even a dead body can be brought to life.

Just about three thousand years back, Shankaracharya had to take help of this knowledge in order to defeat Mandan Mishra in a spiritual debate. But as time passed this knowledge became extinct in the society and today only a very few Yogis have full practical knowledge of this unique practice.

This knowledge is considered to be so important and secret that only a few Yogis, known to me, know of this practice and after them this practice shall perhaps vanish from this earth.

3. Haadi Vidya

This Vidya or knowledge has been mentioned in several ancient texts. On acquiring this Vidya a person neither feels hungry nor thirsty and he can remain without eating food or drinking water for several day at a stretch.

Several Yogis of the Himalayas, remain engrossed in deep Sadhanas for months and years without eating or drinking anything. When they do not eat or drink, they do not even have to empty their bowels. Thus they are able to perform long penance for years and their bodies also remain healthy and fit, even without food. Acharya Vishnu Sarang, the famous Tantrik from Nepal and Yogi Manohar are proficient in this Vidya.

4. Kaadi Vidya

Just as one does not feel hungry or thirsty in Haadi Vidya similarly in Kaadi Vidya a person is not affected by change of seasons i.e. by summer, winter, rain etc. After accomplishing this Vidya a person shall not feel cold even if he sits in the snow laden mountains and shall not feel hot even if he sits in the fire. Thus a Sadhak can perform incessant penance without being affected by change of weather or seasons.

The Jain scholar, Pragya Sun had accomplished both the Haadi & Kaadi VIdyas. Guru Gorakhnath and Matsayendranath too had accomplished them.

Today the Jain scholar of Mahabalipuram Sun Maharaj and Yogi Vishambhar of Badrinath are accomplished in these Vidyas and have kept these practices alive.

5. Madalasa Vidya

On accomplishing this Vidya, a person becomes capable of increasing or decreasing the size of his body according to his wish. Lord Hanuman had miniaturised his body through this Vidya while entering the city of Lanka.

The average height of a human being is six feet. Through this Vidya a person can reduce the size of his body to the size of a mosquito and can even enlarge his body to a size of over hundred feet.

A few years back a conference of Yogis was held on the Bhairav hill, near Dehradun and in this conference Tailang Baba (an ascetic) demonstrated this miraculous practice before hundreds of Yogis. This Vidya is almost extinct today and in my opinion only Tailang Baba has accomplished it.

6. Vayu Gaman Siddhi

Through this Siddhi a person can become capable of flying in the skies and travelling from one place to another in just a few seconds. The Jain scriptures speak of Jain ascetics who could fly from place to place in a few seconds. Swami Divakarsuri and Swami Pragyasuri have been such accomplished ascetics.

About eight years back Vishuddhanandji demonstrated this practice in Varanasi and proved that it is not a myth.

Today Yogi Chaitanya Swami of Madurai and Yogi Niranjan Swami living near Kanya Kumari are the Yogis who have accomplished this practice. But it seems that this knowledge shall perish with them.

7. Kanakdhara Siddhi

One can acquire immense and unlimited wealth through this Siddhi. It's said that once Shankaracharya saw a very poor and destitute woman and with the help of the Kanakdhara Yantra he showered gold in her house. This Yantra is made on a silver plate and 36 squares are formed by drawing 7 lines each, horizontally and vertically. Then the Beej Mantra is written in these squares. Today only a very few people have full and authentic knowledge of this Siddhi.

8. Prakya Sadhan

Through this Sadhana a Yogi can direct his disciple to take birth from the womb of a woman, who is childless or cannot bear children. Several Yogis have thus blessed infertile women with children. Swami Vishuddhanand had accomplished this Sadhana and had used it to bring happiness into the lives of several women. But today only two or three persons are accomplished in this Sadhana.

9. Surya Vigyan

This Solar science is one of the most significant sciences of ancient India. This science has been known only to the Indian Yogis and using it, one substance can be transformed into another through the medium of sun rays.

Swami Vishuddhanand had demonstrated the miracles of this science about 50-60 years ago, by transforming a paper into rose and a cotton ball into gold.

This science has been kept alive by Divyendu Ghosh and some other Yogis, otherwise it has become almost extinct.

10. Mrit Sanjivani Vidya

This Vidya was created by Adi Shankaracharya. Through it even a dead person can be brought back to life. This practice may seem to be a myth but it had been used by Guru Gorakhnath several times. Today only a few persons have practical knowledge of this Vidya.

It is but our misfortune that we consider most of our rich heritage to be just myth when in fact through it we can achieve all success, wealth & comforts in our lives. It's really very shameful that a nation where such unique & distinguished Yogis were born, today, the people of the same nation disbelieve and make fun of their ancestral heritage.

The golden Vidyas which can elevate a human life both materially and spiritually form an indivisible part of the great personality, famous as Poojya Gurudev Narayan Dutt Shrimali.

An ordinary person may feel surprised to know how all these Vidyas can be known by a single person, to such levels, that he has even become capable of imparting it to His disciples. But the scholars having some knowledge of these Vidyas know that Poojya Gurudev is in fact a divine personality more famous as Swami Nikhileshwaranand Paramhans before whom all the Yogis bow down in reverence.

These Vidyas and Siddhis are of very high spiritual level and are not meant to be demonstrated publicly. Today the world is filled with deceit, fraud, violence and greed, hence it has become even more essential to revive and resurrect these divine Vidyas. And to achieve this it also becomes necessary to recognise the true divine form of the personality, who alone is capable of endowing this knowledge on others.

Such knowledge cannot be acquired through books and neither can it be properly explained through this medium. For this a person shall have to become a disciple and learn these rare practices sitting in the Guru's feet. One shall have to come close to the Guru and shall have to give up his position, his ego and all arguments.

I seek the forgiveness of Reverent Gurudev for disclosing this aspect of his personality without his permission. He often says that he does not believe in imparting this knowledge to anyone without testing his faith, devotion and will.

But seeing these ancient Indian knowledges becoming extinct I could not restrain myself from revealing these facts before the readers. I bow down in reverence before Gurudev's holy divine form which is a confluence of so many unique and celestial Sadhanas & Siddhis.

-Yogi Chaitanya Dev

CHAPTER - 14

SADHANA: THE RIGHT WAY

CHAPTER - 14

1. Sadhana : The Right Way

Every Sadhak tries his best to accomplish daily worship and use special Mantra rituals. But every Sadhana has a particular procedure and every deity or the Guru is worshipped in a particular manner: Presenting some important rules is this wonderfully enlightening article.

In every Sadhana, *Upchaar* or special worship of deity has an important place. Upchaar means devotedly making some offerings to the deity in order to win his or her grace.

There is no fixed rule for Upchaar but including this worship procedure in Sadhana assures quicker success. There are different types of Upchaars ranging from Ekopchaar to Sahastropchaar. Our article shall focus only on Shodashopchaar, Dashopchaar and Panchopchaar forms of worship in which 16, 10 and 5 articles are offered respectively. In each age, forms of worship have been different but in the present age of hustle and bustle performing a Sadhana itself is a great fortunate achievement and the shorter the procedure the better.

It is best to do Shodashopchaar worship in which 16 articles are offered but in daily Sadhana Panchopchaar worship would suffice and in it five articles namely fragrance, flowers, incense, ghee lamp and sweets are offered.

2. Shodashopchaar

This includes—

1. Aavaahan
2. Aasan
3. Paadya
4. Arghya
5. Aachamaniya

6. Snaan
7. Vastra
8. Madhupark
9. Tilak
10. Akshat
11. Pushp
12. Dhoop
13. Deep
14. Neivedya
15. Taambool
16. Naariyal

3. Aavaahan

Many do not count this in the procedure and instead just offer prayers to the deity. It means inviting the deity concerned to come and bless the Sadhak. For this both hands are joined and the following Mantra is chanted.

Aavaahayaami Devesh Sarvashakti Shakti Samanvite,
Naaraaynnaay Bhadraay Gururoopaayate Namah.
Guru Brahmaa Guru Vishnnuh Gurudevo Maheshwarah.
Guru Saakshaat Parbrahma Tasmei Shree Gurave Namah.
Aasan

A worship mat is used in order to make the physical body free of ailments, the soul pure and gain divine powers. Basically a man acts as a bad conductor and does not allow energy of Mantra chanting from being earthed. Torn, burnt, and used mats are prohibited. Deer skin, tiger skin, grass, silk, cotton and wool mats are best. Deer skin for gain of knowledge, tiger skin for spiritual progress & wealth, and wool for riddance from sorrows and poverty are prescribed. Deities are offered a mat of flowers and then the following Mantra is chanted.

Ramyam Sushobhanam Divyam Sarva Soukhyakaram Shubham.
Aasanam Cha Mayaa Grihaann Parameshwar.
Paadya

Offering water in the feet of the deity is called Paadya. For this two spoonfuls of water is offered chanting thus.

Yad Bhakti Lesh Samparkat Paramaanand Sambhavah.
Tasmei Te Parameshaan Paadyam Shuddhaay Kalpaye.
Arghya

Water offered to deities for washing their hands is called Arghya. Mix flowers and fragrance in water in a tumbler. Offer chanting thus.

Arghyam Grihaann Devesh Gandh Pushpaakshatcih Sah.
Karunnaam Kuru Me Dev! Grihaannaarghya Namastu Te.
Aachamaniya

Water offered to deities for rinsing the mouth is called Aachamaniya. Offer water chanting -

Sarva Teerth Samaaneetam Sugandhim Nirmalam Jalam.
Aachmyataam Mayaadattam Grihaann Parameshwar.
Snaan

All deities are present in the ocean of knowledge, still three spoonfuls of water is offered as a mark of respect for a bath.

Gangaa Saraswatee Revaa Payoshanni Narmadaajaleih.
Snaapitosi Mayaa Dev Tathaa Shaantim Kurushnna Me.
Vastra

Clean & new clothes are offered. Offering old, torn clothes leads to losses. *Mouli* (holy red thread) can be offered instead chanting thus.

Sarva Bhooshaadi Ke Soumye Lok Lajjaanivaaranne.
Mayopapaadite Tubhyam Grihaann. Parameshwar.
Madhupark

Bathe the deity with honey. The Mantra is -

Om madhuvvaataa Rataayate madhu Ksharanti sindhavah maadhveenrah santvoShadheeh.
madhunaktamutosh so madhumat paarthav (Gum) rajah.
madhu dhaurastu nah pitaa madhumaatro vanaspatih madhumaanastu sooryah maadhvee graavo bhavantunah.

madhu snaanam samarpayaami namah.
After this, bathe the deity again with pure water chanting :
punah shuddhodak snaanam samarpayaami.
Tilak

For riddance from sins, afflictions and misfortune a mark is made on the forehead of the deity. Sandalwood paste is best otherwise Ashtgandh, *Gorochan*, camphor, saffron and musk can also be used. Mantra -

Shree Khand Chandanam Divyam Gandhaaddyam Sumanoharam.
Vilepanam Surshreshtth Chandanam Pratigrihyaataam.
Akshat

Akshat means unbroken rice grains which are offered to gain wealth and prosperity. Mix with vermilion and offer them chanting thus.

Akshtaashcha Surshreshtth Kumkumaaktaah Sushobhitaah.
Mayaa Niveditaa Bhaktyaa Grihaann Parameshwar.
Pushp

Offer flowers to the deity for comforts, good luck and health chanting thus.

Maalyaadeeni Sugandheeni Maalatyaadeeni Veiprabho.
Mayopaneetaani Pushpaanni Grihaann Parameshwar.
Dhoop

Offer incense made from choicest and most fragrant herbs to the deity chanting thus.

Vanaspati Rasodbhootah Gandhaaddyah Sumanoharah.
Aaghreyah Sarvasevaanaam Dhoopoyam Pratigrihayataam.
Deep

Lighting a lamp before a deity signifies dispelling of darkness of ignorance from the Sadhak's life. Mantra -

Suprakaasho Mahaadeepah Sarvatah Timiraapahah.
Sa Baahyaamyaram Jyotih Deepoyam Pratigrihyataam.
Neivedya

Neivedya means elixier. While offering sweets or food articles chant this.

Neivedyam Grihyataam Dev Bhaktim Me Hyachalaam Kuru.
Eepsitam Me Varam Dehi, Sarvasoubhaagya Kaarakam.
Taambool

Offer a betel leaf containing betel nuts, cloves and cardamom. A betel leaf is symbolic of the sixteen *Kalas* or divine virtues. Mantra-

Poongifalam Mahad Divyam Naagvalee-rdaleiryutam.
Elaadi Choornna Sanyuktam Taamboolam Pratigrihyataam.
Naariyal

Take the naariyal in both hands chanting -

yatraa te dhratasy dhrataa te dhaara Ne viniyogah dhee brahraar dhrataa vachanaa yatraasv yatraa bhargo devaanaam dakshi naaye saagarasy mahaalaKshmye sampoor

nayate saprabhaavaan japaa mam tvaam amuk gotrotpannoh ...... amuk sharmaah ...... tvaam purn bal buddhi vidhya purNatvam tvaam charaNe naarikel fal grahmaati tvaam charne samarpayaami namah.

Offer your body, strength and mind to the deity in the form of a naariyal.

4. Neeraanjan Aarti

Sing the *Aarti* (special hymn) of the deity whom you are worshipping. For Aarti use a lamp with one or five wicks. Mantra-

Aanand Matra Makarandam Anant Gandh Yogineendra Susthir Malindam Apaastabandham Vedaant Karannek Vikaashsheelam Naaraayannasya Charannaambuj Maanatosmi.

With this the worship is over. If one is not able to do Shodashopchaar worship one should do Panchopchaar worship while chanting the Mantras with full devotion.

One should daily offer prayers to one's deity and Guru.

Generally, you should perform following rites-

Find out the required direction to sit in for specific Sadhana. Each Sadhana has a specific direction. Then arrange to sit such that you face that particular direction.

1. Place a small wooden board in front of you. Spread a piece of cloth on it. Each Sadhana will have a specific color. Put the photographs of deity, Yantras, rosary and other Sadhana articles on steel plate(s). Unpack the Sadhana articles, if you have received them in plastic packet, and then place them on steel plate(s). Place these steel plate(s) on the cloth-cover on the wooden board. You should not place the Sadhana articles on bare ground. If you do, then all the benefic energy that you gained by performing the Sadhana will get "earthed" and disappear into the ground. If you do not have steel plate, then you may install the various Sadhana articles on the cloth-cover on the wooden board.

1. Always take a bath before starting to perform the Sadhana and then wear the specific color robes. Each Sadhana has a specific color of robes to be worn. In some Sadhanas, your are not allowed to wear any stitched clothes. Men should wear the specific colored Dhoti in the traditional Indian style. Wear the underwear on your body, and then wear the Dhoti. Women should wear specific colored clothes. Wearing Saree (sari) is preferable. The process of wearing saree/dhoti are detailed elsewhere in this faq. You should have received a Guru Chadar/Pitambar (cotton shawl inscribed with Guru Mantra). Wrap this shawl on your upper body below the neck like you would wrap a blanket. Wrap the Guru Chadar/Pitambar (shawl) on your upper body. Don't use perfumes, deodorent or powder etc. Only some Sadhanas (eg. Apsara (Divine nymph) Sadhanas) require you to wear specific flower perfume on body. Do NOT wear shoes/ slippers etc. You should perform Sadhana barefooted.

Find out the details of Prayer Mat/asana (color, texture,type etc.). Asana or Prayer Mat is basically a seat, a piece of cloth. Most of the Sadhanas are performed by sitting on the ground. However, your body should not touch the bare ground. If it does, then all the benefic energy that you gained by performing the Sadhana will get "earthed" and disappear into the ground. Find out the color and type of asana (cotton/woollen etc.). Spread the asana on ground to sit on it.

Each Sadhana has a specific Yogic-asana (sitting pose/posture/ stance) like Padamasan, Sukhasan, Siddhasana etc. Do not confuse this Yogic-Asana with the Asana in above point. A Yogic-asana is a method or Pose/stance of sitting in a specific way. However, as a newcomer in this field, you might not be able to sit in the specific Yogic-asanas or do not know about them. You may sit crosslegged on the asana (on ground) for most of the asanas. You should sit upright with straight back. Some Sadhanas might require to be performed standing up.

Day and Time of starting the Sadhana is very important. You should start the Sadhana at the most auspicious time on the specific day. You may check the auspicious times on our web site here. A time chart for auspicious times is also contained in the Mantra Tantra Yantra Vigyan magazine. Start the Sadhana on the Best time, and then perform it at the same time everyday. You need to check Time only for the first/starting day of the Sadhana. You should be very punctual about the time.

Now, whilest starting the Sadhana, you should light a deepak (lamp) and incense sticks. Place them on the wooden board between the Sadhana articles and yourself. You will need to light either a ghee (clarified Indian butter) lamp or oil lamp depending on the Sadhana. You should always place the Incense in front (in your left side). You should always place the butter oil (Ghee) lamp in front (in your right side). If you are supposed to light lamp with other oils (eg. mustard oil etc.), you should always place such oil lamp in front (in your left side). You should use a cotton wick to light the lamp.

Again, each Sadhana has specific flowers to use. However you may use Rose flowers for most of the Sadhanas.

You will need a small paste of Chandan (sandalwood powder) for the Sadhana. You should add some water to a very small portion of sandalwood paste in a small plate and keep this paste ready.

You should also keep some unbroken rice grains ready for Sadhana near you. The rice grains should not be broken and it is preferable to mix them with some vermilion powder.

You should also keep some fruits ready. Fruits should be in odd number, either one fruit, or three fruit or five fruits.

You should also keep ready a small saucer (preferable a copper tumbler) containing water. Also have a small spoon (preferably copper spoon) ready.

At this point you should light up the lamp and incense. Please ensure to put enough oil/ghee in the lamp so that it keeps burning for the entire Sadhana procedure.

Then, you should start the Sadhana. First, you should take some water in your right palm, and say thus - "Myself (name) son of (father's name) am performing (Sadhana name) on (date) at (time) at (name of place) to (purpose eg. to get riddance from diseases). May I be successful by the divine grace of revered Gurudev. " Then, let the water flow onto the ground. This is a basic agreement between you and Divine done in the presence of natural element (water) to attain success in Sadhana. You should do this on the first day of Sadhana. There is no need to repeat it after that. This is called Sankalp. There is a detailed article on our web site about Sankalp here.

Now, chant the holy word "OM" three times. You should close your eyes and try to extend the chant for as long time as possible whilest breathing slowly. This is done to activate your inner body.

Then, you should mentally meditate on the Divine form of Revered Gurudev in your mind for a few minutes. You should mentally concentrate that you are calling revered Gurudev to come and guide you to accomplish the Sadhana successfully.

At this point, you need to perform some specific rites like welcoming Gurudev (or the deity) and offering them various articles. Detailed Mantras and procedure for this have been printed in various issues of Mantra Tantra Yantra Vigyan magazine. One such good article is "Sadhana : The Right Way" which was published in Mantra Tantra Yantra Vigyan magazine August 2000 issue and is also available on our web site here. A general summary of the main steps in given below.

You should offer some water towards the base of revered Gurudev's photo to wash His feet whilest chanting appropriate Mantra.

Then, you should take some sandalwood paste in the ring finger of right hand, and mark some sandalwood paste on the feet of revered Gurudev whilest chanting appropriate Mantra.. This is done to remove sins, faults, bad luck and tensions from life.

Then, you should offer some unbroken rice (mixed with vermilion) to revered Gurudev on the base of the photograph whilest chanting appropriate Mantra. This is done to get a perfect body, wealth and prosperity.

Then you should mentally meditate that you are offering sweet scented incense made of medicinal herbs to revered Gurudev so that your faults and shortcomings can be destroyed. You should chant appropriate Mantra.

Then, you should mentally meditate whilest chanting appropriate Mantra that you are offering lamp light to revered Gurudev to banish the dark ignorance of knowledge from your heart.

Then, you should offer the fruits to revered Gurudev whilest chanting appropriate Mantra.

Then, you should chant one complete rosary round of the Guru Mantra. The Guru Mantra is

|| Om Param Tatvaay Naaraayannaay Gurubhyo Namah||

You should chant the Guru Mantra using the Sfatik rosary. You should have received it along with your Diksha. This is a white crystal rosary. Details on holding the rosary and chanting Mantra are given elsewhere in this faq. If, for some reasons, you don't have it, then you may use any other rosary to chant the Guru Mantra. Please inform us by email if you did not receive the Sfatik rosary and

Guru Chadar/Pitambar when you applied for Guru Diksha.

You should keep your eyes open and stare with a fix gaze either at the form of revered Gurudev, or the lamp flame. If you perform Sadhana by closing eyes, then there is a possibility of your falling asleep.

Then you should chant the required rounds of the required Mantra with the required rosary. The actual pronunciation of every Mantra is very, very important. If you are in doubt, then you should phone Jodhpur Gurudham to check the correct pronunciation of the Mantra. It is not possible to check the Mantra pronounciation on email/letter, since finer elements like tone etc. cannot be tested. Audio recordings of some Mantras are available on our website here.

Then, you should again chant one complete rosary of the Guru Mantra. Therefore, you should always chant one complete round of Guru Mantra both before and after the required Mantra. This embedding between Guru Mantra is done to increase the beneficial power of your Mantra. If you are performing "Guru Worship" then you should chant at least 4 rounds of Guru Mantra with Sfatik Rosary.

After this, you should mentally pray to revered Gurudev offering Him the complete Mantra chanting and praying for His blessings for success in Sadhana. You should not get up during the entire Sadhana procedure and remain seated upright and erect with straight back. The oil lamp should be burning continuously during the entire Sadhana procedure.

Then, you should stand up. Put the still lighted ghee/oil lamp on a steel plate. Take this steel plate in your hand and sing the Guru Aarti. An English transliteration of the Aarti is listed on our web site here.

After the Aarti, you should sit down and meditate mentally asking revered Gurudev forgiveness for any mistakes (known and unknown) made during the Sadhana process and seeking His blessings for the success.

Then you should bow down in the Divine feet of revered Gurudev.

You should start the Sadhana at the same time daily for multiple days Sadhana. You should always endeavor to complete the Sadhana for the specified number of days. You will start feeling the beneficial effects of the Sadhana after few days of doing the Sadhana. Please ensure to eat only pure, vegetarian food during the Sadhana days and remain celibate (abstain from sex) during this period. Also try to sleep on floor (not on bed) and speak as less as possible (only when required) during this period. Follow other Sadhana related rules religiously.

After the end of the specified days period, some Sadhanas require you to drop the Sadhana articles in water. This is done to give back to nature what nature gave us i.e. to get the required effects from the Sadhana articles, and then to return them back to natural elements. You should drop the articles in the running water (river, stream etc.). While dropping, meditate on the Divine form of revered Gurudev and concentrate that " I am returning the Sadhana articles back to nature. May I achieve full success in my endeavor." After dropping the Sadhana articles in the water, you may continue to do Mantra chanting daily without using the rosary. You cannot reuse the Sadhana articles after dropping them in water. However, if you feel that you have made some mistakes in performing Sadhanas, and/or have not gotten the complete effects of performing Sadhana, then you may repeat the Sadhana upto a maximum of three times with the same Sadhana articles. In this case, you don't need to drop the Sadhana articles after performing Sadhana first time. You may repeat the Sadhana on any other auspicious day. A list of auspicious days for the month is also listed in the Mantra Tantra Yantra Vigyan magazine, and is also available on our website. However, after performing Sadhana three times, you should always drop the Sadhana articles in water.

5. Obstacles For a Sadhak

Back to Issue

It is necessary for a new initiate in the world of Sadhanas not to be frustrated or lose hope by the initial failures. This is a wonderful article for the new Sadhaks which they shall find really heartening and encouraging.

All Sadhanas and spiritual practices have a particular sequence and process. Till all rules are not followed success in Sadhanas remains doubtful. Sometimes success remains elusive to a Sadhak even after hard work. This could be due to the bad Karmas of one's past lives,

Sometimes we also see evil and corrupt individuals earning respect, fame and wealth in life. On the other hand those devoted to the Lord are seen suffering from pain and sorrow. Following are some interesting facts reading which a person could learn low to neutralise past bad Karmas and earn success in Sadhanas.

a. Health

The biggest obstacle to success in any field is bad health. A person can successfully accomplish Sadhanas only when he is perfectly healthy and free from diseases. It is almost impossible to attain to success in Sadhanas through the medium of an unhealthy body. Hence one should be punctual in sleeping, rising, eating etc so that the body could be always fit. Natural healthy food, regular exercise and Yogic postures or *Asans* go a long way in keeping the body healthy.

b. Food

The second obstacle is unhygienic food that not only corrupts the health rather also gives rise to worry and mental disturbance. This is why our ancient texts stress so much on the purity of the food one consumes. There is a saying in the texts - ***Jaisa Ann Vaisa Mann!***

The food one eats determines the purity of one's thoughts. The type of food that one consumes definitely has an effect on one's thoughts. mind, actions. There are said to be three categories of food according to the ancient texts - First category consists of sour, spicy, hot food which is called *Raajasi.* The second category consists of stale food, leftovers, meat and wine called *Taamsik* food.

The third category consists of food obtained through pure means, which is neither too spicy nor too hot. It is called *Saatvik*. It is this type of food that one should eat.

Eating Taamsik and Raajsik food leads to lust, anger, greed, infatuation, arrogance and jealousy. It leads to loss of physical and mental health. Thus a Sadhak could deviate from path of Sadhanas. So one should eat pure and less food.

c. Doubts

The third obstacle on the path of Sadhanas is doubt. When the Guru directs a new person on the path of Sadhanas success is not attained at the very first go.

For example suppose a Sadhak is engaged in an eleven day Sadhana and even by the fourth or fifth day he has no divine experience, then he might be plagued by doubts. Suppose one is doing a Lakshmi Sadhana then during the period of Sadhana the expenses might shoot up. But if one persists and completes the Sadhana then without doubt the Goddess of wealth is pleased and blesses one with financial success. One's stars might have planned a poverty ridden life for the individual and accomplishing Sadhana for wealth would mean fighting against Nature. This struggle could result in a sudden rise in spendings in the beginning. And naturally some Sadhaks might start to doubt the efficacy of the Mantra and the Sadhanas. They might become doubtful whether Gods and Goddesses are actually there or they would ever appear before them. There might be doubts whether t he Sadhana is correct or the Yantra being used is actually Mantra energised. They start to think that if the Sadhana or Mantra were efficacious then the result would have manifested.Because success has not accrued there must be something wrong with the Sadhana or maybe the Guru has guided us wrong. Doubts start to assail their minds and as a result the Sadhak gives up the Sadhana even before he begins it. And even if they do accomplish the Sadhana they do it filled with doubts due to which they are not able to succeed.

Lord Krishna has said in Bhagwat Gita -

Ashraddhyaa Hutam Dattam Tapastaptam Kritam Cha Yat. Asadityuchyate Paarth Na Cha Tatpretya No Iha.

i.e. Havan or *Yagna*, charity, *Tapa* and Sadhanas accomplished without faith and devotion are but useless and they bring no rewards.

Devotion and faith are the biggest assets of a Sadhak. He should have faith in the Guru, in the Mantra, Yantra, gods, goddesses and deities. A real Sadhak should accomplish all Sadhanas determinedly like Lord Buddha.

Ihaasane Shushkayatu Me Shareeram Tvagasthimaansaam Pralayanch Yaatu.

Apraapya Bodham Bahukalp Durlabham Nevaasnaat Kaaymanashchlishyate.

i.e. Lord Buddha had pledged when doing *Tapa* - My body might perish, my skin might shrivel and the bones might crumble but I will not get up from this Sadhana seat till I have had total realisation.

A Sadhak should have such a determination so that he could make actual progress in his Sadhanas. More he progresses more he realises that Sadhanas are not imaginary but real.

d. Sadguru

Sadguru does not mean some human being. Sadguru is an entity who can bestow real knowledge, who can make one rise high in life, who can bestow totality in life, who can direct one to right path.

One needs to reflect on these facts because today there are very few real, experienced and realised Sadgurus. There is no dearth of people claiming to be Gurus. In every street you will find a Guru. But most of them are just arrogant individuals who are only after wealth, fame and physical pleasures. Without having accomplished any Sadhanas they claim to be Yogis and some even call themselves God. In such a crowd of pseudo Gurus it becomes very difficult for a common man to find and choose a real master.

It is the greatest fortune for a disciple to find a Sadguru in his life. A Guru is needed in life to guide the Sadhak onto the path of Sadhanas, to help him overcome obstacles on the path of Sadhanas and to instil divine energy into him in order to overcome problems. The Yogis who are expert in the science of Tantra state that through Diksha obtained from a Guru a Sadhak gains divinity and all his sins are absolved.

Changing Gurus frequently also leads to problems in Sadhanas. Although all Sadhanas lead to the same goal yet the paths are different. Today you might start *Prannayam* and tomorrow on advice of some other person you could take to *Hatth Yoga*. Third day you might even give up Yoga and start chanting some Mantra and fourth day you might take to listening to divine discourses. Wandering from one path to another or changing Gurus cannot help one make progress.

Lord Krishna has said in Gita -

Tad Viddhi Prannipaaten Pariprashnen Sevayaa. Upadekshyanti Te Gyaanam Gyaaninas-tatvadarshin.

i.e. To gain real knowledge go to those who have realised Supreme Element. By bowing before such Yogis, by serving them selflessly, by asking them questions sincerely one can learn a lot. These are means to please them and then they become willing to impart true knowledge.But this knowledge can be gained only from a Sadguru.

e. Fame

One big obstacle for a Sadhak on the path of spiritualism is fame. When people living around realise that a Sadhak has successfully accomplished a particular Sadhana they become devoted towards him. They start to give him regard through their words and gestures. The Sadhak too is but a human being and he too likes to be respected and honoured. When he gets these from the society he starts to crave for more and more. As a result he forgets his aim of worshipping the Supreme and joins the race of earning more fame and name. This results in loss of Sadhana power. He loses his innocence, humility and becomes arrogant. Purity of mind and heart is lost and one is filled with anger and false pride. So a Sadhak should never reveal his powers to the society. One must rise high in the spiritual world and not in the material world. This is the real way to progress.

f. Celibacy

Another obstacle on path of spiritualism is sex. Until there is enough energy in Sadhak's body he cannot succeed in Sadhanas. One needs power of the physical body, mind, senses and soul and this energy is conserved and boosted through *Brahmacharya* or celibacy. Hence a Sadhak should not indulge in excess sex. He should shun negative company and not eat food that could delude the senses and lead to loss of celibacy.

Even the married Sadhaks should observe celibacy as much as they could, to preserve vital energy. More one restrains oneself more the energy that builds up and faster one succeeds in Sadhanas.

Lord Hanuman remained a celibate throughout life and as a result he had immense physical strength. He was brave, powerful and very spiritual. He was most devoted to the Lord. He possessed all knowledge and all divine powers called *Siddhis*. It was due to these powers that he could assume a giant form or become smaller than even a fly. When crossing the ocean on his way to Lanka he assumed a huge form and jumped over the ocean. And when entering Lanka in order to avoid being detected he assumed a form smaller than a fly.

Bheeshma observed celibacy throughout life and as a result he was blessed with the power that death would not come to him till he so desired. Lord Parshuram who was invincible and who had defeated everyone on earth had to face defeat after a battle of 23 days with Bheeshma. This was the result of the celibate life Bheeshma led.

g. Wishes

The Sadhak who does not become free of material wishes has to face many obstacles on the path of Sadhanas. Wishing and desiring leads to anger, infatuation and greed and as a result the Sadhak loses his balance of mind. Hence once should always keep the mind free of desires.

h. Criticising others

Finding faults in others is the biggest obstacle for a Sadhak. A Sadhak should not waste his time in such activities and not worry what others are doing. The Sadhak should always remain concentrated in his own Sadhanas so that there is no time left for such useless activities.

Those who fall into habit of criticising others cannot progress well in Sadhanas, for they are wasting a lot of their thought power in a useless exercise. One should always remember the words of the great saint Kabeer -

Buraa Jo Dekhan Mein Chalaa, Buraa Na Miliyaa Koy. Jo Dil Khojaa Aapanaa, Mujhasaa Buraa Na Koy.

i.e. When I started to look for bad qualities in others I ultimately realised that there is no more bad person than me.

Remember that if you point one finger at others in accusation three fingers shall be pointing towards you. What I mean to say is that before accusing others even once evaluate your own self at least thrice. One should look at one's own thoughts and try to remove one's faults instead of finding the same in others.

CHAPTER - 15

TANTRA: THE LEFT-HAND PATH OF LOVE

CHAPTER - 15

1. The mysterious Tradition

This article attempts to outline, in an extremely general way, some basic ideas of the Tantric tradition. Even though the author has a rich personal experience in some of the practical aspects of TANTRISM, the intention here is not to expose a personal view, but to present the Tradition in its most pure form, without any kind of "western interpretations" that most of the time kill and destroy the authentic meaning. This is done with the sincere intention to revive, mostly from the practical point of view, this lost Tradition and to reveal the true face of TANTRA Science.

2. A unified theory of Consciousness

YOGA and TANTRA form the primitive lode of the Indian spiritual tradition, a foundation deeply connected to universal philosophies. Much has been written and discussed regarding these studies, but due to their profoundness and hidden symbolism they remain opaque. A secret throughout the centuries, TANTRA remains diffuse, mysterious and puzzling yet constantly present in the diversity of yoga techniques, especially in its Tibetan forms. With purposeful investigation, it presents a genuine science of man where cosmic forces mingle with physiology, psychology, magic and spiritualism. TANTRA offers a practical, multi-leveled vision of the human being, a unified theory that explains the most intimate aspects of man's behavior which have evaded current research. A detailed, sincere study and practice of TANTRA would contribute to the enrichment of contemporary science and psychology in a manner not as yet conceived.

3. A Way for our Age

The disciplines of TANTRIC schools recognize in Kundalini the source of a mysterious energy an energy still not properly defined by modern science but of paramount importance for a complete spiritual emancipation. If we add that the Ageless Wisdom defines TANTRA as the spiritual system best adapted to our era of KALI YUGA, where spirituality is declining even as man and woman are desperately trying to reintegrate themselves into a creative and spiritual cosmic center, we realize the significance of these techniques. Today we are bound to an "objective" knowledge which is becoming more and more mechanical and inhuman. Abstract thinking is linked less and less to real life yet defines most of our activities. Therefore, it is absolutely necessary to practice TANTRA, a highly accurate, subjective knowledge which is accessible to everyone, through experience and verification.

4. The web of Love

The ultimate purpose of all forms of yoga is to indicate the way to fully integrate into the Objective Reality and realize an harmonious merging into the different levels of the phenomenal cosmic manifestation. The main goal is to always act in perfect concordance with the harmony and superior cosmic activity. This is why, through different yoga techniques, the practitioner's consciousness is expanded and the superior perception aptitudes are amplified and developed to the utmost. These characteristics are common to all systems, TANTRA YOGA being no exception.

TANTRA envisions the Universe as an extremely complex, multidimensional web of invisible energies. This Science permits the controlled expansion of consciousness beyond the web of illusory appearances and thus liberates us from ignorance. TANTRA is also called VAMA MARGA, i.e. The Left Hand Path, due to the fact that women, who are of lunar influence, negative polarity or the left, play an essential role in this Science. However, The Way which is recommended here is not at all made of negations or austerities as in most other spiritual systems, but of pleasure and beatitudes. TANTRIC tradition puts forth clearly that the state of harmonious integration and spiritual freedom can be obtained only through direct experience and living of everyday life. The inferior levels of consciousness cannot be efortlessly controlled and surpassed unless fully and frantically, intensely and totally, lived in the whole plenitude of their power.

5. The Way of pleasure

In this respect, TANTRIC texts say that nobody will be able to obtain spiritual perfection using difficult and boring techniques. Perfection can be realized easily using the fulfillment of all wishes. The very same processes that for others could cause decay or death, venom or evil, can be used wisely and firmly for spiritual uplifting and transformed into a miraculous cure of the soul.

"One can fall due to the earth, another one can, without doubt, raise himself with the help of the earth." (Here "earth" is symbolic of woman and creative energies.)

Another text says:

"If a man is a YOGIN, he does not enjoy sensual pleasures; while one who enjoys them cannot know YOGA. That is why the KAULA (a TANTRIC School) way, containing the essence of sexual enjoyment and YOGA, is superior to all paths. In the KAULA approach, sexual enjoyment turns into YOGA directly. What in conventional religion is considered sin becomes meritorious." KULARNAVA TANTRA 2. 23

In the TANTRIC tradition, YOGA (union with God) is simultaneous with the passionate living of worldly delights, leading to the state of enlightenment through the supernormal powers (SIDDHIS), which are obtained through practical application of these special procedures. These powers serve a definite purpose in the way of attaining the Supreme.

6. The human Temple

TANTRA YOGA considers that the human body, with all its biological and psycho-mental processes, is only an instrument in which and through which the cosmic forces operate. The individual human structure and the outer macrocosmic manifestation, or Universe, are similar. Therefore all that exists in the Universe should also exist in a certain form and proportion in the microcosm, i.e. the human body.

7. Sanctified Sexuality

The TANTRIC philosophy itself includes in its theory all the levels of the Universe and gives a paramount importance to astronomy, biology, parapsychology, anatomy, meditation, medicine, music, art and even sexuality. In fact, the sexual experience, considered to be a unification of the Everlasting Male (+) and Everlasting Female (-) principles, has a very important place in TANTRIC techniques and procedures which are often profoundly erotic.

TANTRA is a complex discipline, an accurate method and a profound analysis based on rational foundations, it is a Meta-Science dealing with the different aspects of the Supreme Consciousness and ways to experience it. Here, sexuality forms only the basal, prima facie of its techniques. It is subjected to a rigorous discipline, because it is known that the secret of Life lies in controlling the sexual energy.

To understand the TANTRIC attitude toward sexuality requires a totally open mind and a reversal of perspective. Accustomed as we are by a puritanical mentality to seeing sexuality as a "sin" to be avoided and ashamed of (or, in any case, to keep it "secret" because of its "impurity"), we have all the chances to consider TANTRIC Love as being a defiant assault on conventional morality and thus to miss completely the tremendous spiritual value of such a perspective. In order to understand it, we must first come to view the human dimension as vibrating in identity with the sacred, divine aspects of Creation. From this sacred perspective, sexuality is seen as re-producing at a smaller scale the continuous and beatific interaction of a Cosmic process which is manifesting the entire Universe from the Absolute Reality. In this new vision, "sin" disappears (it never existed, anyway!), being replaced by pure beatitude and total love. Sexual union is thus a form of meditative discipline with profound psycho-mental and spiritual effects.

Therefore there is no obscenity or pornography but only sublime symbolism and refined beauty. The figure of a man and woman coupled in sexual union is not thought impure or sinful. On the contrary, it is considered to be a veritable sacrificial rite. The male worshipper has an attitude toward the woman which is different from that of an ordinary person performing the sexual act. The woman is transfigured into a living symbol and earthly manifestation of the Divine Mother of the Universe (PARA SHAKTI). Likewise, for the woman, man represents a vital embodiment of the Everlasting Male Principle (SHIVA). The sexual beatitude raised at the transcendental level of an extraordinary psychic experience with a spiritual character reflects, then, the ineffable happiness of a subtle cosmic nature, known in YOGA as ANANDA (i.e., cosmic beatitude) and in TANTRA as SAMARASA (i.e., the savor of equality).

8. Returning to origins

TANTRA YOGA considers that the human being has an extremely complex body and mind. The usual consciousness of wakefulness is considered to be only a very small fraction of our native intelligence, fruit of a very long period of evolution and development of the human being. The practitioner tries to follow the same road of evolution but in an opposite direction. He must go through all stages in inverted order and leave them behind, until he finds the starting point or the unique origin. This is logical if we realize that TANTRA considers the human being to be a summary of the Universe and therefore all the cosmic elements have their correspondent in the visible and invisible man.

9. The Diamond Body

Consequently, the TANTRIC way does not mean to run away in an alienating foreign spiritual universe, for the TANTRIC practitioner wants to take with him in his evolution all the structures of his body creating in this way the famous "diamond body," (VAJRAYANA) which is beyond the limitations of time. The transformations that take place then consciously free all the potential of the human being. This has a positive repercussion on the body, considered as a unitary whole composed of visible (i.e. physical) and invisible (i.e. subtle) structures. Yearning tirelessly to grasp the enigmatic silence and the fascinating mystery of the Cosmos, the TANTRIC practitioner becomes an integral part of this mystery in the bosom of which he absorbs and identifies himself. For this, the external practice and the internal mutation are both indispensable because they make it possible to understand within themselves (through identification or SAMYAMA) the phenomena, leading to an authentic and sometimes ineffable understanding of the cosmic forces that surround us. Modern scientists are still making weak attempts to decode them, but for the TANTRIC practitioner these subtle forces are everyday realities.

10. Everything is Light

For example, using the techniques of MANTRA (subtle attuning sounds) meditation, the TANTRIC masters discovered long ago that there is an objective rapport between sound and light. For them, light is just a sound of a certain frequency. The visible appearance of every object is due to a concentration and simultaneous reflection of the light. This multiple reflection lowers the frequency of the energy which then crystallizes in physical forms. Light frequencies are seen as different colors. Sound and color are related in the same way as are life and form. Every color corresponds to a certain sound and vice-versa; every sound has its subtle energetic color-form. A MANTRA is a subtle mental sound that facilitates the attuning to the mysterious frequencies of the cosmic forces. When a MANTRA is uttered correctly (UCCARA), its color-form starts to manifest also in a degree that depends on the nature and intensity of the uttering.

11. SHIVA and SHAKTI

In the TANTRIC philosophy, every letter of the Sanskrit alphabet is a BIJA MANTRA (seed sound) which is associated with a certain part of the human body or, to be more specific, to a certain petal of the power centers (CHAKRAS). This shows that the different parts of the human body are the manifestations of the different dynamic aspects of an Essential Energy known in TANTRA as KUNDALINI SHAKTI, an enigmatic and complex subtle power which lies in a latent form at the base of the spine. TANTRA YOGA considers that the Ultimate Truth is easily attained through the beatific union of PURUSHA (the Spirit) and PRAKRITI (the Nature); or, in TANTRIC terminology, through the union of SHIVA and SHAKTI. SHIVA represents the pure passive Consciousness, the static aspect of the Ultimate Reality. SHAKTI is the creative power of the Universe, the dynamic feminine element, the matrix of endless possibilities through which the Infinite and Unique Consciousness can manifest.

12. Relationships release Power

Any profound fusion of the complementary opposites, or reintegration of polarities into the origins of the whole, automatically brings a breakthrough into higher levels and leads to a gradual re-discovery of primordial spontaneity and unity (SVATANTRYA). This transcendency of opposites is a transcendency of the Cosmos because this movement abolishes the duality. The frantic and complete embrace of SHIVA and SHAKTI merges them forever in a Unique Principle. And in the bosom of the Ultimate Reality reached in this way, there is no more SHIVA or SHAKTI, there is only UNITY, there is only ONE. All physical, biophysical and psycho-mental aspects of the Cosmos return to this Unity which emanates and reabsorbs them continuously.

13. The Life Chain

Life is ONE; all its forms are in a mutual relationship within the bosom of an extraordinarily complex and infinite WHOLE. Any kind of action from the part of any being, must automatically, through reflection, influence any other form on the same level of creation. We are but links of an infinite chain. We are made of the same substances as that of stars and galaxies. We have inside ourselves the same energies and powers as the ideal Gods have. They lie only dormant, ready at any time to be awakened and used.

14. The Universe—Illusion or Reality?

Consequently, the TANTRIC practitioners engage themselves in a continuous process of self-discovery and of discovery of the Universe at the same time. They ask themselves: "Do we see and perceive the world the way it really is or only the illusory appearance? And in the last case, are we condemned to see forever only this illusory appearance, without ever attaining the Essential Reality?" If a person could perceive the fourth dimension through the special capabilities which lie dormant in every human being, his or her vision of a stone, for example, would be completely different from that of an ordinary person. More than that, a TANTRIC practitioner who attains the state of absorptive meditation (SAMYAMA) on the stone could see, feel and even hear the energetic vortexes of the apparently invisible electrons of the stone.

15. Seeing with the eyes closed

In this respect, TANTRA claims that we must detach ourselves from all external forms in order to fully perceive that which the veil of illusion (MAYA) hides, and only then can we discover the Ultimate Reality and realize the complete freedom from the painful chains of ignorance. Only by closing our eyes can we have an authentic vision. In the ultimate act of vision, the body, i.e. the totality of the energetic and physical structures of the human being, meditates exactly as the spirit does. The very old treatise TANTRA TATTVA says that only the man who sees everything as being within himself sees the Truth. The Unknown and the Mysterious surround us everywhere, inside and outside ourselves. Realizing this, the TANTRIC practitioner must resort to the perfect, practical knowledge of the subtle energies which are latent in every human being and which can be awakened through proper techniques. These energies are the vehicle for the Spirit, freeing it from the hallucinating shadows of ignorance. In this new state the human body becomes the modality of experimentation and of return to the primordial Androgynous unity—the Lost Paradise.

16. Experimental duplication

TANTRA Science relies upon the practical realization of its teachings. Here we are not dealing with endless talking and argumentation but instead with engaging ourselves fully and thoroughly in an exceptional practice which can lead the practitioner to Freedom, Pure Existence, Super-Consciousness, Beatitude and supernormal powers (SIDDHIS). The SAHITYA TANTRA advises, “Start the practice under the surveillance of a TANTRIC initiate. If, after a certain time, you do not obtain any positive results, then you are free to quit.” In the same way that benefits can be obtained only by using a remedy, the truth of the TANTRIC Science can really be proved only through successful practice. However, it is necessary to stress here that the TANTRIC practitioner develops and perfects his SIDDHIS only for the purpose of raising himself at the level of the Supreme Being and from there to fuse eternally with the Absolute. The SIDDHIS have no value per se; they are only a modality. But all these powers cannot be obtained by only talking about TANTRA, for tireless practice and direct experimentation only can lead to such unusual achievements. About this, there is no doubt.

17. The Libido—thirst for Unity

Another aspect which is important in TANTRA YOGA is that the libido, when manifested as sexual drive, is not at all considered to be only sensuality but, at the innermost levels, as the soul's ardent yearning for spiritual perfection. Here the erotic impulse appears as the psyche's abyssal thirst to reach perfection through unity of complementary polar opposites. In this way, re-born as a genuine Androgyne of the Secret Tradition — magical child of SHIVA and SHAKTI — the Individual Spirit will have access to the highest levels of Consciousness. The magnetic Woman, the electric Man TANTRA considers that, energetically speaking, woman is magnetic, passive, lunar, receptive and charged with power of negative polarity (YIN). In multiple ways, she attracts, absorbs and stores subtle energy which remains latent. When connected in a proper way with the male electric, dynamic and positively charged subtle energy (YANG), the female energy undertakes a complex alchemical reaction and thus the couple generates an energetic power station. This is very easy to verify. Certain TANTRIC techniques enable the practitioner to verify that the bioenergetic differences of polarity between man and woman are energized to the highest extent through the love play and that a mutual exchange between these two forms of energy (YIN/female, YANG/male) takes place during sexual intercourse in which the two partners harmonize themselves on multiple levels. Performed in the TANTRIC way (successive orgasms without ejaculation) these unions can intensify and develop the latent extrasensorial capacities and the mental power of both partners beyond any expectations.

The couple who practice TANTRIC sexual union use the subtle energies of the man's body and the complementary energies of the woman's body for attaining the state of harmony with the Absolute.

18. Retention—the untold secret

It is important to emphasize that TANTRA YOGA substantiates its techniques of spiritual development on the perfect yet efortless control of the sexual energy (semen retention). Traditional texts say semen contain consciousness as the ova contains primordial creative energy. Here the point is to return to the practitioner the enormous amount of raw sexual energy contained in semen and in the correspondent female orgasmic emanations in such a way that this subtle energy may be sublimated and its efficiency used for higher purposes, i.e. psycho-mental and spiritual.

Being in perfect physical, emotional and mental health is a must for approaching any of the sexual practices of TANTRISM. Modern civilization leaves integrity, so we need to open up and to re-learn to experience as intensely as possible our senses. While it is true that cultivating the sensory awareness, here being included different techniques of amplifying the sexual pleasure and of opening up to experience deep sexual orgasm, can be a useful preparation for TANTRA, these incipient techniques are not TANTRA yet if they are not accompanied by a total, yet effortless, control.

The Science of the ancient Sages (SIDDHAS) teaches that the sexual reproductive power (the Life Force) can be transmuted into superior forms of energy called OJAS and TEJAS. The practitioner causes his seed to rise up to his crown center (SAHASRARA), where it becomes transformed into SOMA, the Nectar of Immortality. Through the TANTRIC procedures, the semen is took over by the lymphatic system. The lymphatic system consists of the fluid (lymph) that bathes the tissues, being similar in composition with plasma. The lymph contains white cells involved in the immunity system of the body. These white cells produce antibodies, special substances which attack the foreign organisms (microbes, etc.) and render them harmless. Through the lymphatic system, the semen reaches the brain (CORPUS CALLOSUM) where it is processed into extremely subtle energies (OJAS and TEJAS) used by the higher mind. As the physical brain needs oxygen and proteins to function properly, the higher mind (superconsciousness) needs big quantities of OJAS and TEJAS energy. The TEJAS energy is that energy which produces the halo around the saints' head. The OJAS energy is that energy which confers an extraordinary vigor, power and virility.

The transmuting of the semen's energy into OJAS and TEJAS does not take place only in men. Women who practice TANTRA YOGA realize the transmutation of that energy which produces the ova and the menstrual cycle. These energies are transformed into OJAS and TEJAS exactly as in the men's case. As a result, the menstrual cycle becomes scarce or even disappears completely, and the ovulation process slows down or even stops. Nevertheless, when the conception of a baby is desired, the energies are permitted to accumulate at the pelvic area, the ovulation returns to normal and the menstrual cycle appears again.

19. The magical spring

In TANTRA YOGA, one uses sexuality for completely transcending it. Even at the level of ordinary sexual experiences, the couple sometimes has the strange and powerful feeling that sexual intercourse releases a tremendous energy inside the human psyche. Frequently superior and nostalgic truths can be inferred in this state. Pedro McGregor in his famous PSYCHOSEXUAL SYNTHESIS confirms the TANTRIC teachings concerning sexuality. Our burning sexual or emotional beatitudes are nothing other than a degenerated mysterious enthusiasm. Our highest and noblest spiritual yearnings, the whole of our transcendental and sublime potential, would be somehow imprisoned in matter, i.e. in sexuality. This enthusiasm is materialized, therefore limited, absorbed and inert. It is logical to consider that a conscious change in our sexual behavior and in our most intimate attitudes could act as a magical spring, releasing truly super-human energies in the same way that a controlled mutation in the intimate structure of the atom can release a tremendous amount of nuclear energy.

20. The energy of intense emotions

Therefore, another important characteristic of the Tantric Way is that spiritual growth is realized through extreme intensity of energy (SHAKTIPATA) spontaneously born during the frantic living of intense emotions, including both sexual and non-sexual emotions. The Supreme Existence reveals itself instantaneously during the tumult of violent emotions such as extreme terror, vivid curiosity, deep compassion, total anger, profound pleasure.

"In order to penetrate into the Supreme Reality, everything that is at hand is to be considered as a modality; because, as the TRIKA system puts it, the human being must not submit to any restrictions (in order to attain the Supreme)".
A tantric text by ABHINAVAGUPTA

When controlled and directed by a lucid mind, this paramount intensity of the extreme emotions creates the instantaneous welding of all levels of the human being (physical-sexual, emotional and mental-spiritual) which are normally disconnected and therefore acting independently. Thus, the practitioner becomes aware of the inner abyssal power that lies within himself and starts to bring it to the surface. The transcendence of the inferior levels of consciousness is realized through an exceptionally frantic living of every moment of everyday life. In this way, the duality disappears into the flashing unity of the Supreme Consciousness, without change (NIRVIKALPA).

21. Why sexuality?

In the act of lovemaking the couple embodies the dyadic wholeness of the Supreme. TANTRIC sexual union resonates with the very foundational energies of the Universe: it captures, magnifies and re-directs the essential Cosmic Power of Life. It is therefore not by chance that sexual intercourse brings the most intense emotional experience that the human being can have while in the flesh. Therefore TANTRA uses it predominantly to create that overwhelming unifying energy. The erotic impulse stirs up the KUNDALINI energy so that it can rise, through the subtle duct of power along the spine, to the highest center of power above the head. This process renders the adept immortal:

> *"Loss of semen is loss of power. Exposure to sexual stimulation arouses this power; controlled the power is like steam in a boiler, no longer random."*
>
> *"The YOGIN who can protect his BINDU (semen), overcomes death; because death comes by discharging BINDU, and life is prolonged by its preservation." HATHA YOGA PRADIPIKA, III, 87*
>
> *"BINDU is under the control of the mind, and life is dependent on BINDU. Hence, Mind and BINDU should be protected by any means." HATHA YOGA PRADIPIKA, III, 89*

In this vision, intercourse becomes a genuine cosmic process at the level of the unified microcosms of the couple, who tries to reproduce the cosmic union of SHIVA and SHAKTI, i.e. of Consciousness and Energy.

> *"In YAMALA or VIRA-YOGINI tradition [Tantric schools], there is physical union (SAMGHATTA) between VIRA (the male) and YOGINI (the female). The purpose is only to stimulate NITYA-ANANDA (the eternal beatitude) by means of the contact of the sex organs. This contact gives intense delight [for the body and spirit]. A text by ABHINAVAGUPTA*

In this sacred act a savant analogy intervenes where physical postures (ASANAS), gestures (MUDRAS), colors, sounds (MANTRAS), musical rhythms and perfumes blend to create a paradisiacal environment. Thus, intercourse serves a purpose much superior to that of sensuality. This precise analogical correspondence leads to a profound intermixing between the level of the chaotic multiplicity in which we live and the Unique Macrocosmic Reality. Through frantic super-sensual fusion of the subtle complementary principles, man and woman realize the alchemical sublimation of the sexual energy. This phenomenon, which leads to a gradual liberation from the painful limitations of Space and Time that restrain terrestrial life, propels man and woman towards the cosmic ecstasy (SAMADHI).

22. A double purpose

As stated before, ejaculation, identified with the sudden loss of this propelling spiritual power, is completely contrary to the attainment of beatific bliss. The violent explosion of ejaculation and of correspondent female orgasmic discharge acts at inner levels as a harmful release of vital subtle fluids and represents a serious loss of power, making it impossible to use the purified sexual energy (OJAS). Therefore the spiritual ascension is immediately stopped. This is why all TANTRIC treatises put forth the necessity for man and woman to control and even completely eliminate ejaculation. Here, the purpose is double: to retain seminal fluid (conserve energy and achieve higher states of sexual pleasure, enabling the man to fully satisfy his woman and himself) and to transmute its energy (acquire magical power and achieve expanded levels of consciousness). The effect is cumulative.

23. Breath, thought and semen

For this purpose, at peak moments, the couple's attention must be focused to simultaneously control the breathing (by making it calm and relaxed), the mind (by focusing it upon a unique object) and the semen (through rhythmically contracting and relaxing the pelvic floor muscles). This procedure acts simultaneously upon the three basic levels of the human being — the physical, the emotional and the mental — creating a perfect harmony between them. Thus, sexual intercourse becomes a genuine love meditation.

24. "Stay with the fire of the beginning"

The most recent conclusions of modern sexology agree with traditional TANTRIC teachings. Sexual therapists are starting to encourage couples to focus more on the process of lovemaking rather than on the end result, i.e. ejaculation. A TANTRIC treatise says:

> *"Stay with the (erotic) fire of the beginning and avoid the poison of the end."*

The satisfaction found in this way is incomparably greater than having an ejaculatory orgasm. The most revolutionary conclusion of the sexual researchers is that man doesn't need to ejaculate at all when making love to a woman. The fundamental error couples make, due to ignorance and bad habit, is to believe that ejaculation and orgasm is one and the same thing and that ejaculating is the peak pleasure for a man and woman. There is nothing more false.

25. Orgasm and ejaculation

Stated with extreme simplicity, orgasm is an intensely beatific state of consciousness and canceling of ego, with profound harmonizing, relaxing and regenerative effects. Male and female ejaculation is only a complex physiologic process of explosively energetic discharge with a dim manifestation of a brief, incipient orgasm, experienced in a selfish unilateral way. During ejaculation, the energy is quickly wasted and for no purpose (except when conception is wanted).

26. The choice is yours

The most important differences between an ordinary orgasm with ejaculation and TANTRIC successive orgasms without ejaculation are illustrated in the following comparative analysis:

ORDINARY ORGASM (with ejaculation)

TOTAL SUCCESSIVE ORGASMS (without ejaculation)

Explosion (outward-bursting energy). Inevitably, the erotic energy is lost permanently and uselessly. The intensity of a following sexual act diminishes greatly compared to what was felt at the beginning. Implosion (inward-burst ing energy). The erotic energy sublimates and is transmuted in ever more refined forms of energy which are gradually accumulated in the depths of our being, producing extremely refined and intense states of pleasure and expanded consciousness. The intensity of the following sexual acts increase constantly and do not diminish in the end.

Lasts a very short time, creating a nostalgic state of frustration due to the partial lack of fulfillment (especially for women, who need a long time to reach the peak of excitement). Beyond time, lasting indefinitely therefore is contiguous with Infinity. Ocean-like state of beatific fulfillment felt by BOTH man and woman as a shared feeling of happiness and joy of living which expands the perception of pleasure. The two lovers become gradually aware of the God(dess) within. Man can share woman's multi-orgasmic capacity without losing the erection.

In the physical body only. Inside as well as outside the physical body, in the subtle invisible body and in the surrounding environment. All beings and objects seem to make love at the same time.

Playing with the other. Playing within yourself with a simultaneous, telepathic perception of the other through empathy, "I feel the other as if he/she is myself."

Dependency. Independence. The other "disappears" due to the spontaneous transfiguration. Both man and woman expand endlessly their merged consciousness into the Universe.

Woman passive/man active. Woman active/man passive.

Heavy breathing. Easy, calm and quiet breathing.

A reflex or instinctual act leading to loss of control, an unconscious, animalistic, irrepressible experience. Hyper-conscious and fully controlled act leading gradually to ecstatic, erotic abandon and happiness which lasts as long as two to three days after a successful TANTRIC experience.

Chaotic movement. Non-movement followed by slow wavelike movements to which the other's body answers tenderly and insatiably in a perfect harmony.

Limited sexual availability due to the exhaustion which follows ejaculation. This leads gradually to a state of permanent fatigue and drowsiness which can manifest as instinctive repulsion for the other or as lack of self-esteem. Unlimited sexual availability making possible an overwhelming erotic experience of a paramount intensity which can last eight to ten hours without interruption —providing that BOTH man and woman perfectly CONTROL the sexual energy. The erotic vitality of the couple amplifies leading to a clear state of inner power and of complete sexual fulfillment.

Fear of undesired pregnancy. The use of contraceptives has many unhealthy side-effects such as hormonal imbalances leading to obesity. Complete freedom of any restrictions or fears. Because of the total semen retention irrespective of the duration of the sexual act, pregnancy is out of the question when undesired. Man becomes a completely safe lover and his woman will never have to use contraceptives when she makes love with him. This leads to a totally natural birth control.

Attachment, selfish desire, possessiveness and jealousy. Detachment, desire transcended into fulfillment, leading to a state of peace with oneself and of tender happiness which overflows to other human beings as love and compassion.

Due to the huge loss of sexual energy, the sexual experiences become less and less fulfilling and, through a reflex mechanism, the psycho-mental potential decreases. Due to the complete transmutation and sublimation of the sexual power, the psycho-mental potential is increased leading to the awakening of paranormal powers (telepathy, clairvoyance, etc.). A state of overwhelming euphoria grows gradually, opening the couple to positive, affectionate feelings. Dramatic increasing of vitality leading to the shortening of the need for sleep and awakening of the creative imagination and lucidity. Man's virility and woman's pluri-level multi-orgasmic capacity awakens and amplifies to the highest extent, leading to ever more fulfilling sexual experiences.

The dynamics of the couple decreases with time and desire transforms quickly into habit. Monotony kills the desire and the relationship becomes ever more trivial. The dynamics of the couple is enriched every day with new and amazing discoveries of the other's inner world and, through reflection, of one's own inner profile. Desire transforms gradually into genuine and pure love, a feeling rarely known by humans and which grows constantly, fed with new and unexpectedly delicious experiences. Habit cannot survive due to the hyper-intense and spontaneous living in the ever-changing present.

27. Conclusion

In TANTRA, sexual union is one of the possibilities offered to man and woman to concentrate and direct the consciousness's activity toward the Supreme Being. Due to the enormous intensity of this union, the consciousness of both partners develops and fuses, at the beginning between themselves and later with the Cosmic Consciousness. The indescribable beatitude then felt embraces all things and beings. All that still subsists is a never-ending thirst for unity, only a Lover and a Loved-one.

TANTRA is a genuine and exceptional form of YOGA which puts sexuality in its right place, recreating the missing spiritual dimension of the sexual experience. This practice expands the human consciousness to the greatest extent and considerably enriches the knowledge of Man and the Universe. At the same time, through the surprisingly links established among apparently heterogenous phenomena and scientific facts, TANTRA opens the road toward infinite horizons, where many extraordinary discoveries wait for the tireless practitioner.

CHAPTER - 16

YOGA NIDRA

CHAPTER - 16

1. Yoga Nidra

Many people in the East and the West are attracted to Yoga Practices, for they think they can find solution to every problem therein, be it physical, mental, emotional or spiritual! A great importance is attached to relaxation techniques that might help a person tensed due to chronic stressful life style. Yoga Nidra is one such wonderful technique, not only for physical or mental relaxation but also for preparing the mind for spiritual discipline, concerning mainly with pratyahara (withdrawing senses form sense-objects) and dharana (concentration). It is to be understood that sleep is not relaxation, for tensions cannot always be resolved completely in ordinary sleep. Yoga Nidra is qualitatively different relaxation. It is a 'sleep' where all the burdens are thrown off to attain more blissful state of awareness, a relaxation much more intense than ordinary sleep. As Swami Satyananda Saraswati (Preface to "Yoga Nidra", 1982, Bihar School of Yoga, Monghyr, Bihar, India) says: 'When awareness is separate and distinct from *vrittis* -mental modifications, when waking, dream, and deep sleep pass like clouds, yet awareness of Atman remains, that is the experience of total relaxation. That is why, in *Tantra*, Yoga Nidra is said to be the doorway to samadhi!'

2. Neuro-physiologic Basis

There is no question about the close relation between the and the brain. Various centers in the brain control, modify, and affect our bodily functions. In fact, there is a center in the brain for every act, whether willful or reflex, physical or mental. Experimental data have identified many such specific centers. Stimulation of these centers leads to appropriate actions, be they motor or sensory, secretary or emotive, affective or cognitive. Thus we have a holographic representation of on the brain. To put the thing more concretely, it is proved that the left half of the is represented in right half of the brain and vice-a-versa. As far as the muscular actions are concerned, the representation is in an 'upside down manner' in motor area of pre-central gurus. Thus, at the top of this part of brain the lowest portion of our -foot- is represented. Then comes ankle, leg (calf), knee, thigh, hip, trunk, shoulder, arm, elbow, wrist, palm, fingers, thumb, then neck, jaw, face, eyes, ears, tongue, taste, swallowing, etc. The same thing is applicable for sensations. Stimulation of brain centers of sensory cortex evokes sensations on the opposite half of the body.

3. Yoga Nidra Practice

In Yoga Nidra exactly opposite process is used to make the brain centers active by focusing awareness on the parts of the in a definite sequence. Thus, the person tries to stimulate various parts of the brain by focusing the awareness on the corresponding parts of the body. By awareness is meant 'attitude of witness' towards physical or mental actions of the body.

4. The Technique

Usually it takes from twenty to forty minutes to complete one Yoga Nidra session. The procedure is carried out by first doing a few *asanas* -practicing a few postures. Then the person lies on his or her back in totally relaxed posture (shavasana -posture simulating dead body). Eyes are lightly closed, arms are kept with palms facing upwards and fingers are half lifted from the ground, breathing is natural and quiet.

5. Resolve or *sankalpa*

Before the rotation of awareness the aspirant should make a positive resolve about the aim in life. The wordings should be clear and precise. It is not expected that the sadhaka makes minor resolves like, 'I will give up smoking, or drinking, or tobacco, but he or she should think higher. A few resolves are:

a) I will awaken my spiritual potential,
b) I will be successful in my all undertakings,
c) I will achieve total health, Or
d) I will a positive help in spiritual progress of others, etc.

i. Rotation of Awareness

Then the rotation of awareness begins. Patient has to just visualize the part of the mentioned by the instructor, be that a teacher or a tape-recorder. The student must not move any part of his body. Quickly corresponding with the instructions, he or she has to shift his or her awareness from one part to the next. The aspirant should not imagine the next part before the instructor mentions it. The whole process is a pleasure and not a burden. There should not be any anxiety or expectation.

The usual pattern is to start focusing awareness in the following sequence:

First on the right side:

The thumb, fingers (one by one), palm of the hand, then the wrist, the forearm, the elbow, arm, shoulder, right back, hip, thigh, knee, leg, ankle, foot, great toe, other toes of the right foot.

The same sequence is repeated for the left side.

Then awareness is focused on the proximity of with the carpet (ground). Back of the head, shoulders, back and spine, thighs, heel. Next the front of the surface is brought in to awareness. Face, brow, eyes, nose, lips, mouth, ears, chin, neck, chest, abdomen.

ii. Awareness of the breath

After rotation of the consciousness in such a sequence, focusing attention on the act of breathing completes **physical relaxation**. One simply maintains awareness of breath, either at the nostril or of its passage through the navel and throat. It is claimed that the process, in addition to concentration, assists pratyahara from the subtle in subsequent processes.

iii. Feelings and Emotions

Next comes **relaxation at the level of feelings and emotions**. Attempt is made to bring to memory the intense physical and emotional feelings; they are re-experienced or re-lived and then effaced.

Usually this is practiced with pairs of two opposite feelings like hot and cold, lightness and heaviness, pain and pleasure, joy and sorrow, etc. Relaxation at the emotional level and building up of strong willpower are the two major outcome of this procedure.

iv. Visualization

The final stage of yoga nidra relates to **mental relaxation**. The aspirant tries to visualize the objects as described by the instructor. Usually such images and symbols are chosen that have universal significance. To quote a few, such as mountain, river, ocean, temple, church, cross, saint, flower etc.

The practicc helps to develop self-awareness and helps in concentration - dharana. Rarely, even meditation -dhyana- may be the natural outcome.

v. Ending the practice

Once again the resolve or *sankalpa* is intently thought of or even visualized. Thus, consciously one tries to direct the unconscious mind about the goal in life. This time the unconscious is very receptive and therefore, may accept the suggestion from the conscious mind with more intensity. It is claimed that in due course of time, depending upon the sincerity and regularity of the sadhaka, the resolve bears fruit in sadhaka's life.

vi Utility

Yoga nidra helps in restoring mental, emotional, and physical health by way of relaxation, and makes the mind more conducive to pratyahara -withdrawing senses from thier objects, dharana -concentration, and meditation. Such a practice helps harmonize two hemispheres of the brain and the two aspects of autonomous nervous system viz. sympathetic and parasympathetic. The impressions in the subconscious are brought to surface, experienced and removed. Thus, the fixation of awareness to the is replaced with awareness linked with subtler aspects of prana and spiritual dimensions. *C S Shah.

CHAPTER 17

The therapeutic psychology of 'The Tibetan Book of the Dead'

By Robert Wicks

CHAPTER - 17

Although we usually conceive of death as the endpoint of life, there is an important sense in which death, as an aspect of change and renewal, is ever present throughout life: each passing moment "dies" as it becomes past experience; a new moment is constantly "born" as the future becomes present. From moment to moment, beginnings and endings perpetually coincide. At a more mundane level, we also frequently meet with another form of death—a counterpart to our familiar conception: our habitual patterns of expectation and reaction to circumstances often lead to a deathlike stagnation and unanimated redundancy within our experience. This narrowing of horizons, though certainly problematic, does not preclude the permanent possibility of experiencing a liberating transformation of character and a "rebirth" of personality. The implicit and explicit means to achieve such a personal transformation within our present lives, as described in The Tibetan Book for the Dead,[1] is the subject of this essay. My aim is to recall and reemphasize some of the affinities between the text's therapeutic intentions and the goals of psychotherapy, in recognition of its practical, socially all-encompassing message. In the course of this inquiry, I will discuss how some authoritative commentators on the text, namely Carl Jung and Lama Anagarika Govinda, have drawn our attention away from the text's more pragmatic and existential value as a handbook for more insightful and liberated living.

In ordinary practice, The Tibetan Book for the Dead is read aloud as part of a Tibetan Buddhist funeral ceremony: it speaks to the dead person who, as a disembodied spirit, is believed to persist within hearing distance in an after-death realm of transition, or bardo. This is a transitional realm through which a disembodied spirit passes between reincarnations.[2] The text's manifest purpose is to offer the dead person repeated opportunities for enlightenment during the bardo experience, such as to avoid rebirth into a renewed condition of suffering. This transitional experience, most importantly, presents itself as a period of decision making: the dead person can choose either to become enlightened by giving up his or her "unconscious tendencies" that inevitably led to suffering, or the person can choose to remain bonded to those dispositions and become fated to circle once more through the patterns of his or her former existence. The text's guiding words are intended to help the dead person choose the path toward enlightenment. On the face of things, then, the text articulates the mechanisms that cause a disembodied soul to gravitate toward reincarnation, and be directed toward the avoidance of suffering through an enlightening personality transformation.

The after-death experiences described in The Tibetan Book for the Dead begin with those immediately following bodily death, and end with experiences that occur just before the disembodied person is reborn into a new physical body. The initial after-death experiences are moments of perfect clarity and insight. These are short-lived, however, and soon fall off into partially enlightened modes of consciousness, which themselves eventually degenerate into increasingly hellish and horrific experiences of bewilderment, selfishness, and animal aggression. The latter, absolutely terrifying, states of consciousness arise as the disembodied consciousness, after having failed to forsake its unconscious tendencies time and time again in its descent through the stages of the bardo, approaches the moment of being reborn into a new physical body and the world of ordinary life. Though couched in religious terms, the text's underlying message is familiar and commonsensical: people who do not change their ways are fated painfully to repeat themselves.

Since the after-death states of consciousness range from the heavenly to the hellish, individuals of different personality types will see themselves reflected in one or another of the bardo states. If one is a relatively enlightened person, then one will feel akin to the visions within the more peaceful bardos; if one is a more violent and selfish person, then one will easily recognize the visions within the more hellish after-death states. The text assumes that no one to whom it speaks is a perfectly enlightened personality, so at each stage of the after-death experience, the dead person receives therapeutic advice on how to overcome his or her "unconscious tendencies," whether the tendencies involve ignorance in general, overwhelming desire, envy, jealousy, or aggression. At whatever level of mentality the dead person is at home, the text aims to release the person from the confines and sufferings that characterize that individual's particular psychological condition.

The manifest contents of the after-death states of consciousness are visions of various Tibetan gods and demons. These deities appear to be as "real" as life within the after-death experience, but the text instructs the disembodied consciousness to regard them as merely the dream-like reflections of its own inner self. The gods and demons can thereby be viewed as symbolic forms expressive of the disembodied consciousness' basic psychic tendencies. In this respect, The Tibetan Book for the Dead is a psychological document that characterizes basic personality styles and presents the principles of those personalities in a symbolic and condensed, yet fantastically realistic, manner.

The key instruction that, if acted upon, generates a liberating personality transformation is repeated at each level of after-death consciousness: whatever the contents of the particular bardo phase happen to be, the disembodied consciousness is instructed to regard the objects experienced within that phase as nothing more than its own psychological projections. The assumption is that upon seeing one's own godlike or demonic reflection as having no more substance than the moon's shimmering image in a pool of water, the natural attachment to one's egocentered personality will soften. By interpreting the godlike and demonic objectifications of one's personality as illusory, one will be able to see one's own individuality itself as illusory. In this way, forsaking one's egocentered self-conception leads to enlightenment. With this issues an elimination of personal suffering, since suffering is believed to be caused by egocentric forces such as ignorance, pride, jealousy, envy, and desire—forces that are objectively embodied by the godlike and demonic visions. Regarding these deities as "empty" entails a recognition that the psychological forces that generate personal suffering have no substantial reality.[3]

The exposition above broadly characterizes the manifest purpose and meaning of the text—a meaning that recognizes after-death states of consciousness, images of gods and demons, and rebirth into a new material body either as a human or as some other form of sentient creature. Complementary to this manifest meaning, however, is a more symbolic meaning—one that reveals how The Tibetan Book for the Dead is pragmatically and existentially directed toward the "dead" who are still living, and not especially toward those who are clinically dead. To reveal this less obvious meaning, we need to examine more closely some of the key features of the manifest meaning, for these indicate that both the existence of gods and the existence of an after-death bardo realm are questionable.

With respect to the reality of the gods and demons that are experienced in the after-death state, we have noted that the text informs the disembodied consciousness that these deities have no substantial reality of their own. Indeed, this is the central illuminating principle of the text. Two memorable excerpts are as follows:

> Through the instruction of his guru he will recognize them [the visionary deities] as his own projections, the play of the mind, and he will be liberated. It is just like seeing a stuffed lion, for instance: he feels very frightened if he does not know that it is really only a stuffed lion, but if someone shows him what it is he is astonished and no longer afraid. So here too he feels terrified and bewildered when the blood-drinking deities appear with their huge bodies and thick limbs, filling the whole of space, but as soon as he is shown he recognises them as his own projections or as yidams; the luminosity that arises later,

mother and son, merge together, and, like meeting a man he used to know very well, the self-liberating luminosity of his own mind spontaneously arises before him, and he is self-liberated.[4]

> [W]hatever you see, however terrifying it is, recognise it as your own projection; recognise it as the luminosity, the natural radiance of your own mind. If you recognise it in this way, you will become a buddha at that very moment, there is no doubt. What is called perfect instantaneous enlightenment will arise on the spot. Remember![5]

These excerpts confirm that the gods and demons experienced in the after-death state, although they appear with a reality equal to the material objects in the world of the living, are indeed believed to be nothing more than manifestations of the dead person's own psychological states.(6) They are merely symbolic forms that express conditions of either psychological liberation or psychological bondage and suffering. This suggests that the path to enlightenment in no way depends upon favors or obstructions issued from the realm of the gods and demons that populate the after-death state; the path depends upon initially recognizing the images of the gods as manifestations of oneself in various possible and actual forms. Self-recognition alone initiates the path to more satisfactory levels of consciousness. Although emotionally powerful in its employment of metaphors like the image of the moon and the recognition of a fearsome lion as merely a stuffed animal, the text's key instruction for enlightenment rests upon a questionable line of reasoning.

To see this, we can distinguish between the form and the content of the visions of gods and demons within the bardo. Their form is to "look real"; their content is the disembodied consciousness' individual personality structure. With regard to the deceptively realistic form of the visions, although the dead person might feel vaguely at home within one of the bardos, it is not initially obvious to the dead person that what is being experienced is simply a projection of himself or herself, and not some objective realm of gods and demons.

The situation is comparable to a person, who asleep in the midst of a vivid dream, remains unaware that he or she is only dreaming. What key instructions do is wake up the dead person to the true nature of the experience, such as the dissolving of the objective form of the experience. When the visions are seen as they truly are, they are appreciated as having no independent reality and hence no power over the dead person, as would be the case if they existed independently. Revealing that the realistic appearance of the bardo visions is deceptive, however, does not entail that the psychological content expressed by these visions is itself illusory. If the objects in a dream, for example, are shown to the dreamer to be none other than a figment of his or her imagination (e.g., as when one teaches a child to see that the objects of a nightmare are simply imaginary), it does not follow that the psychological structure that that dream objectively presents is also a figment of the imagination. For example, an imaginary monster within a young child's nightmare could very well express the child's inner anxiety. So from the recognition that the objects of the bardo experience are illusory, we cannot also conclude that the individual self that projects these objects is itself illusory. Such an individual self may indeed be illusory upon further reflection and in consequence of further argument, but this does not itself follow from the recognition that the dream-like visions have no substantial reality of their own.

These considerations lead us to examine another aspect of the dead person's dispositions of character or "unconscious tendencies" that the gods and demons symbolically express. Representative of the more enlightened states are buddha forms that embody the fusion of compassion and knowledge; representative of the more animalistic states are flesh-eating demons, who, screaming "strike" and "kill," tear corpses limb from limb. With respect to interpreting the text in a practical and existential manner, it is important to determine whether there is good reason to interpret these represented states of consciousness literally, as after-death states occurring in an actual, after-death bardo, or whether it makes more sense to regard the after-death bardo itself as another projection of consciousness. If the latter is the case, then the after-death bardo would indeed represent a transitional condition, but one that can occur only within living experience. It would also follow that the consciousness that projects the after-death bardo could be none other than that of a living, flesh-and-bones person.

It might be thought that a definitive interpretation of the after-death bardo realm, either as a literal or as a purely symbolic realm, would depend upon how the text characterizes the essence of consciousness. We shall see, however, that the description of the essence of consciousness within the text is logically independent of whether or not there are actual after-death states of consciousness. In view of this independence, it remains well within the text's overall spirit to interpret its references to the after-death bardo as purely symbolic and, hence, as potentially quite meaningful to those who cannot recognize an afterlife. This, as we shall see, characterizes Lama Govinda's view, although he arrives at this perspective through a different line of reasoning. Before considering his interpretation, though, we should briefly examine how the text describes the essence of consciousness, and note that this description neither implies nor precludes the existence of after-death states of consciousness.

In its description of the experiences immediately following death, The Tibetan Book for the Dead characterizes consciousness as it is in itself. This is the condition of consciousness that is regarded as the ground of all experience. We can consider three alternative translations (1927, 1975, and 1994, respectively) of a central passage:

> Thy breathing is about to cease. Thy guru hath set thee face to face before with the Clear Light; and now

> thou art about to experience it in its Reality in the Bardo state, wherein all things are like the void and cloudless sky, and the naked, spotless intellect is like unto a transparent vacuum without circumference or centre.[7]

> As soon as your breath stops, what is called the basic luminosity of the first bardo, which your guru has already shown you, will appear to you. This is the dharmata, open and empty like space, luminous void, pure naked mind without centre or circumference.[8]

> Just as your breath stops, the objective clear light of the first between will dawn as previously described to you by your teacher. Your outer breath stops and you experience reality stark and void like space, your immaculate naked awareness dawning clear and void without horizon or center.[9]

These passages assert that at the point of death, the dead person initially experiences the true, "clear and void" nature of consciousness—a "luminous emptiness" or "shining void." Soon thereafter, the dead person loses contact with this, the person's own universal nature, and begins to experience more idiosyncratic objectifications of himself or herself in the form of godlike and demonic projections—projections that reflect the unconscious tendencies of his or her personality. The experiential movement of the book, understood literally, is thus from a universal and liberated consciousness that appears to present reality in itself, to more and more particularized and restricted forms of consciousness, which represent the limited reality of the dead person's egocentricity. These latter forms do not represent consciousness in its purity, but consciousness as "karmically obscured" in its more familiar, benighted, and bewildered forms—ones that we can recognize as typical of ordinary consciousness. Although the text states that the gods and demons experienced in the after-death states are the projections of the dead person's consciousness, the excerpts above still leave indeterminate the status of consciousness as a "luminous void." It could be that, although the gods and demons are illusory, that the experience of the "luminous void" is not. On the other hand, it could be that the experience of the "luminous void" as representative of an actual after-death state of consciousness is also an illusion. There are thus two questions to be distinguished:[10] should a reasonable reading of the text recognize any after-death states of consciousness at all?[11] if it is reasonable to recognize after—death states of consciousness, which, if any, reveal either consciousness as it is in itself or reality as it is in itself? The manifest meaning of the text suggests that there are after-death states of consciousness, and that only the experience of consciousness as "clear and void" is truly revelatory. It remains unclear whether what is revealed is the nature of consciousness independent of the nature of reality or the nature of consciousness as nature of reality, but the spirit of the passages suggests the latter.

Consistent with the key passages cited above are two alternative positions:[12] reality is consciousness, and this is immediately known when consciousness is in the state of luminous emptiness during this life and/or during the initial after-death bardo state;[13] reality in general is indeterminate or indeterminable, but the reality of consciousness in itself, whatever its relation to reality in general happens to be, is a luminous emptiness. Both of these alternatives are consistent with the existence of after-death states of consciousness; both are also consistent with the nonexistence of after—death states of consciousness. With regard to the second of the alternative views above, some further explanation may be appropriate, since one might believe that the claim that "all reality is consciousness" entails the existence of after—death states of individual consciousness. This, however, would not follow. There need not be after-death states of an individual's consciousness (i.e., a dead person or "ego" who has after—death experiences), since at the moment of actual bodily death it is possible that every individual consciousness completely, and without a moment of personal reflection, dissolves into the universal consciousness, just as a raindrop dissolves into the ocean.

From an analysis of the text's explicit claims about the nature of consciousness, then, we are left without a definitive position regarding the actuality of after-death states of consciousness that a dead person, as such, might experience. That is, if we accept that consciousness is essentially a luminous void, this alone does not imply the existence of after-death states of consciousness. We must subsequently approach the latter issue from a different angle, for example through an inquiry into the universality of the states of consciousness described in the after-death realm. It is safe to assume that anyone who lives and dies in a place communicationally dissociated from Tibet in either time or space (e.g., ancient Peru) is not likely to experience Tibetan Buddhist gods in an after-death state of consciousness. Even supposing, quite remotely, that such a person had after-death experiences of the kind described by The Tibetan Book for the Dead, the entire symbolic meaning of the gods—a meaning revealed to the dead person by exposure to The Tibetan Book for the Dead—would be virtually meaningless.[14] This fact alone goes very far in leading us to question the universality, not to mention the very reality, of the after-death visions of gods and demons described in the text. If, however, we were to acknowledge the existence of after-death states of the very general kind that the text describes, then perhaps a plausible position would be to maintain that after one dies, one experiences a series of basic human personality structures in some symbolic form or other.[15] Without some guide to the experiences, though, there would still be little possibility for salvation or enlightenment. The possibilities for the dead person's enlightenment depend so heavily upon the instructions given in The Tibetan Book for the Dead, or upon some comparable text or person who can fully communicate these instructions, that without such guidance, the person will regard the symbolic forms as realities, and not as projections of his/her own personality. Moreover, there remains the issue of whether there is indeed any communicational interface at all between the world of the living and the world of the dead, let alone one that can be crossed simply by means of inspired vocalization or mental concentration.

Such complications suggest that it is more reasonable to interpret the text as directed more toward the living than toward the dead, and directed more toward psychological realities than toward metaphysical ones. This leads us to regard the text mainly from a psychological and therapeutic perspective. Quite consistent with this is the essential spirit of Buddhism as a practice-centered, and not speculation-centered, outlook. Chandradhar Sharma describes this well:

> [Buddha] repeatedly told his disciples: "Two things only, my disciples, do I teach—misery and the cessation of misery." Human existence is full of misery and pain. Our immediate duty, therefore, is to get rid of this misery and pain. If instead we bother about barren metaphysical speculations, we behave like that foolish man whose heart is pierced by a poisonous arrow and who, instead of taking it out whiles away his time on idle speculation about the origin, the size, the metal, the maker and the shooter of the arrow.[16]

Buddhism in general issues from the perception and experience of suffering in this world of the living, and is grounded upon fundamental prescriptions to alleviate this suffering. Given this pragmatic emphasis at the core of Buddhist insight, it would be consistent to interpret The Tibetan Book for the Dead as predominantly written for the "dead" of this world—those whose lives are tangled within cycles of desire, jealousy, envy, hatred, and aggression that generate continual suffering. This would include everyone at one time or another during their lives. The existence of suffering within this life is an absolute certainty; the existence of after-death states of consciousness is a matter of speculation and interpretation.[17] It is commonly said that The Tibetan Book for the Dead is a book for both the dead and the living. The present interpretation suggests that it is certainly a book for the living, and perhaps one for the dead.

If we consider The Tibetan Book for the Dead as certainly a book for the living and maybe one for disembodied souls, then Carl Jung's authoritative and respected psychological commentary on the text stands in need of re-evaluation.[18] This is not because Jung acknowledges the existence of an afterlife; it is because his psychological interpretation draws the reader away from those very parts of the text that address living people who now suffer. This as we shall see in a moment, is partly the result of Jung's interest in showing how his own psychological theory fits the text more comprehensively than Freud's.

Before considering the details of Jung's psychological commentary, it is important to note why either Jungian or Freudian psychology is compatible at all with the spirit and meaning of the text. This has been alluded to above, and arises from the very close affinity between the character of ordinary dream consciousness and the after-death experiences described in The Tibetan Book for the Dead. It is well known that both Freud and Jung interpret dreams as symbolic of fundamental psychic contents. According to Freud, these contents are basic sexual tensions; according to Jung, they are universal thought structures, or "archetypes." Independently of the accuracy of Freud's or Jung's views on the specific nature of dream contents, both believe that although the items experienced within any particular dream have no objective reality of their own, they nonetheless symbolically reveal the psychic nature of the person who dreams. Similarly, with the possible exception of the initial experiences of the "luminous void," the after-death states of consciousness described in The Tibetan Book for the Dead are understood to represent symbolically the nature of the dead person's individual personality, as represented by deity-like objectifications of his or her "unconscious tendencies" - tendencies that lead the person into cycles upon cycles of rebirth and suffering.

This affinity between ordinary dream states and the after-death states of consciousness described in The Tibetan Book for the Dead establishes a close connection between the Western practice of psychoanalysis and the Tibetan Buddhist concept of rebirth: successful psychotherapy entails a rebirth of personality. The goal of psychoanalysis is to improve an individual's psychological health by revealing to the individual that individual's basic psychic structure and constellations of inner conflict. Within Freudian and Jungian analysis, this structure is discerned through an examination of the person's dreams (among other methods), since dreams are regarded as the symbolic manifestations of the person's psychic energy. The Tibetan Book for the Dead comparably aims to bring an individual into a condition of increased psychic health (i.e., enlightenment) by displaying the individual's "unconscious tendencies" symbolically and objectively, such as to allow the individual subsequently to render these forms ineffectual within his or her psyche. For example, if an individual is angry and violent, the text powerfully and shockingly illustrates the world of angry and violent people for the individual to contemplate, and then urges the individual to reinterpret that world as akin to no more than a reflection in a pool of water (i.e., as illusory). The procedure aims to dissolve the meaning and reality of the individual's former world by detaching the individual from involvement in that world, and by allowing the person thereby to become "reborn" into a more enlightened condition as a new personality. In these basic ways, both the psychoanalytic method of dream interpretation and the modes of visionary interpretation and liberation expressed in The Tibetan Book for the Dead aim to alleviate psychic suffering and to restore mental health. Both are fundamentally therapeutic in their inspiration and aims.

In his psychological commentary to The Tibetan Book for the Dead, Carl Jung points out how the text first describes the highest stage of consciousness in the experiences immediately after death, and then goes on to describe more and more animalistic forms of consciousness. Addressing the Western reader, and intending to offer a more familiar orientation toward the text, Jung offers a "reverse" reading that begins with the more common states of consciousness and gradually progresses toward the more enlightened states. Reconceptualized in this way, the series of bardo experiences forms an ascending path reminiscent of the Christian conception of spiritual development—a path that begins with imperfect and finite humanity and extends toward a perfect and infinite God.

Dante's Divine Comedy would clearly exemplify this conception, as it begins with a description of hell and then progresses to descriptions of purgatory and heaven.[19] Complementary to his intention to provide the Western reader with a more familiar orientation toward the text, Jung urges a "backwards" reading for the purpose of contrasting his psychological theory with Freud's. Near the very end of the after-death experience (which Jung reads as the "beginning"), the text most intriguingly describes the psychological effects of assuming a specifically male or female identity: the assumption of a male identity generates love for one's mother and aversion toward one's father; the assumption of a female identity generates love for one's father and aversion toward one's mother. Since The Tibetan Book for the Dead was composed as early as the eighth century A.D., quite independently of the development of Western psychoanalysis, these observations offer some startling confirmation of Freud's core insights into the development of sexual identity.

Rather than wholeheartedly acknowledging that The Tibetan Book for the Dead confirms Freud's insights, jung points out that the sexual attitudes noted by Freud originate and operate only within what the text describes as the most primitive and unenlightened form of consciousness (i.e., in ordinary, day-to-day consciousness). Jung takes this as evidence that, with its strong emphasis upon sexuality, Freud's psychological theory penetrates only into the elementary layers of the psyche. He adds that when we progress to the less instinctual, and more enlightened, conditions of consciousness, we reach levels that are better comprehended by Jung's own theory of archetypes.

Due to Jung's orientation toward higher levels of consciousness and his interest in criticizing Freud's psychological theory, his commentary on The Tibetan Book for the Dead has the subtle effect of leading the reader away from the text's vivid descriptions of the less enlightened forms of consciousness. The problem with this approach, however, is that it fails to recognize that almost everyone, at one time or another, lives within these more animalistic stages of sensual pleasures, sexuality, and desire, and that by downplaying the text's prescriptions for overcoming psychic bondage within such conditions, one undermines the potentially widespread effectiveness of the text's practical application.

As a handbook whose intention is to reveal the path to enlightenment to the great majority of those who are now alive, The Tibetan Book for the Dead speaks to the large audience of individuals who must start along this path from one of the lower realms. The text itself acknowledges that only a mere handful of people—those who have practiced meditation their entire lives—end their life in a highly refined and illuminated psychological condition. Since most people do not live with a consciousness of this sort, there is an important sense in which the basic orientation of Jung's interpretation is implicitly counterproductive: it draws our attention away from that part of the text that speaks to most people. This suggests that reading the text from its natural beginning is the most appropriate way to experience the work: the reader begins with a description of the ideal, enlightened state of mind, and gradually descends into more and more hellish conditions until—if one is a typical person whose daily consciousness is informed with reports, and perhaps experiences, of wars, sickness, poverty, and crime—one encounters a reflection of one's daily world of ignorance, envy, jealousy, and violence mirrored near the end of the book. The experience of reading the text in this way indicates to the reader exactly how far he or she actually is from an enlightened condition, and allows the reader to interpret his or her present condition (assuming that the person is in a condition of ordinary consciousness) as the culmination of many levels of spiritual loss. Such an experience of self-recognition is exactly what the text intends to generate in its readers.

Similar to Jung. Lama Anagarika Govinda offers a psychologically centered interpretation of the text. The following excerpt summarizes his view:

> The different bardos, therefore, represent different states of consciousness of our life: the state of waking consciousness, the normal consciousness of a being born into our human world, known in Tibetan as the skyes-nas bardo; the state of dream-consciousness (rmi-lam bar-do); the state of dhyana, or trance-consciousness, in profound meditation (bsam-gtan bar-do); the state of the experiencing of death (hchhi-kha bar-do); the state of experiencing of Reality (chhos-nyid bar-do); the state of rebirth-consciousness (srid-pa bardo). All this is clearly described in The Root-Verses of the Six Bardos, which together with The Paths of Good Wishes, from the authentic and original nucleus of the Bardo Thodol, is that source around which the prose parts crystallized as commentaries. This proves that we have to do here with life itself and not merely with a mass for the dead, to which the Bardo Thodol was reduced in later times.[20]

Lama Govinda interprets the text as referring primarily to "different states of consciousness of our life," and in this respect his account is directed toward the living, and less toward disembodied spirits. At the same time, though, we can ask how many of the living are taken into consideration within his view. This question arises because Lama Govinda's attitude toward the text's essential meaning is clearly aristocratic: he refers to the text's true meaning as accessible only to "initiated disciples" in Tibetan meditative practice. Although he regards the text as a psychological document—as "a key to the innermost recesses of the human mind"—he maintains that this "key" is far from accessible to everyone:

> Only he who has ears to hear, i.e., who has prepared himself in life for the call of liberation and has made himself receptive for it by training his inner organ of hearing, can respond to the call and follow it. Only he who has opened his inner eye can see the redeeming visions. Those, however, who have neither developed the faculty of inner hearing nor that of inner vision, cannot be benefited by merely listening to the recital of the Bardo Thodol.[21]

As does Jung, Lama Govinda interprets The Tibetan Book for the Dead in a way that draws our attention away from its generally applicable therapeutic aspects. He directs our attention toward the more enlightened states of consciousness, but precludes the experience of these states to all but the properly initiated. Insofar as only a small group of people practice Tibetan meditation, the true meaning of The Tibetan Book for the Dead will, in his opinion, remain a "secret" doctrine.[22]

The Tibetan Book for the Dead may indeed contain subtleties of meaning that are accessible only to those who have practiced Tibetan meditation for decades. To privilege this level of knowledge as the essential meaning of the text, however, leads one's focus away from the less enlightened states of consciousness—those states of consciousness that are typical of the majority of the human population. Just as Jung downplays the more instinctual and bewildered states of consciousness due to his interest in revealing the limit of Freudian psychology, Lama Govinda, due to his keen interest in the meditational experience of higher states of consciousness, similarly focuses our attention on the more elevated and more inaccessible states of human awareness.[23]

The prevailing spirit of The Tibetan Book for the Dead, however, opposes aristocracy and elitism. It is clearly a book addressed to everyone, independently of the reader's capacity for profound insight or abstraction. The book offers a series of opportunities and procedures for achieving enlightenment, such that if one fails to comprehend the path to enlightenment at one level, then one receives another chance at another level. The book begins by addressing the most receptive people, and tells them simply to consider their experiences in a certain way (namely to regard their experiences as the result of their own psychological projections).

If they can do so, then enlightenment follows. If the text's instructions are impossible to follow with such ease, then the reader moves into a less enlightened condition and receives the same instructions as before, with some added incentive. Sometimes more gods appear to assist the person, with the hope that the increased social presence of the gods will cause the person to adhere to the text's directives. If this effort to enlighten the person again fails, then the same message is introduced once more, except that it is accompanied by more and more terrifying imagery. At some level of consciousness, it is hoped that the person will finally achieve the awareness to interpret his or her world in a more enlightened way. At every level of consciousness, then, there is a prescription for enlightenment. At every level of consciousness it remains possible —if only the correct mode of interpretation were to be adopted— to spring instantaneously into an enlightened condition.[24] The following passage unequivocally displays this socially all-encompassing interest of the text:

> Up to now there have been seven stages in the dangerous pathway of the bardo of the peaceful deities, and by being shown at each of the stages, even if he has not recognised at one he will have at another, and boundless attainments of liberation occur. But although many are liberated like this, sentient beings are great in number, bad karma is very strong, the neurotic veils are heavy and thick, the unconscious tendencies last for a long time, and this cycle of confusion and ignorance neither wears out nor increases, so there are many who are not liberated but wander downwards, although they have been shown accurately in this way.[25]

Addressed here is a far more widespread audience for The Tibetan Book for the Dead than is emphasized by either Jung or Lama Govinda. Both interpret the text convincingly in their efforts to understand its profound psychological import, but in terms of the text's function as a therapeutic tool to lead any person to enlightenment, independently of whether that person is intrinsically closer or further from an enlightened condition, Jung and Lama Govinda offer interpretations that leave most suffering people behind.

The Tibetan Book for the Dead is a book written especially for benighted and bewildered souls. It acknowledges that enlightenment is difficult, and that it takes many repetitions of the key message for there to be any significant spiritual effect. It repeats its message that we, and only we, are the source of our desires, our interpretations, our evaluations, our pleasures, and our fears, and that we can render such sources of suffering ineffectual, if we were only to interpret the apparent seriousness and significance of the world as the play of our own creation. In this respect, The Tibetan Book for the Dead is a book of practical wisdom comparable to Epictetus' Handbook; it offers a set of advisories intended to reduce suffering and to guide all people, not just the select initiates, toward a rebirth of personality and composure—a rebirth to take place not within a life after clinical death but within our very present life.

NOTES

1. Although the English translation of the Bardo Thodol (The great liberation through learning in the bardo) has been titled The Tibetan Book of the Dead, it is not quite a book "of" the dead, but rather a book "for" the dead. Since the latter is more aptly descriptive, I will refer to the Bardo Thodol as The Tibetan Book for the Dead throughout this essay.

2. In Robert Thurman's translation of the text, the bardo is simply referred to as "the between." See Robert A. F. Thurman, trans., The Tibetan Book of the Dead (London: Aquarian Press, 1994).

CHAPTER 18

Tantric Sex - A Spiritual Path Of Ecstasy

By Swami Nostradamus Virato

CHAPTER - 31

At a time when even the word "sex" is suspect, it is vitally important to explore the depth of this misunderstood phenomenon from a new perspective...a spiritual one.

We came into this body through the act of procreation...better known as sex. Unless you were artificially inseminated, you wouldn't be here unless a man and woman had sexual intercourse. They had it because it gave them animal pleasure drawn by a deep spiritual pursuit. While we are in a body, this pleasure underpins much of our lives. It matters not if you are a nun, monk or prostitute. Whether you deny it or not, sex runs much of your existence. Unfortunately most of us have lost that special ingredient of this physical attraction that moves us beyond mere physical pleasure to a deeper and more satisfying wholeness.

At one time, long before so-called civilization permeated our culture, humans cultivated this pleasure to transcend into higher dimensions of consciousness, beyond the material, animal orgasm. Thousands of years ago, people had achieved a high degree of awareness and an alchemical formula for converting what we know as sex energy—called by many names such as Chi, vital force, soul, etc.—using it to enter into a state of Divinity. Their spiritual philosophy held sexuality as a divine rite and an expression of union or yoga.

Unfortunately, as our planet moved out of the Taurien Age (4300-1700 BC) and became masculine and aggressive, it also lost this deep spiritual connection to this vital sex energy. While sexuality touches every part of our lives, it's sad that this most pleasurable life-affirming phenomenon—the act of creating our very birth—is today tainted with fear, abuse and general negativity.

There was a time when people with an awakened consciousness practiced Tantra with an artistic and cultural lifestyle of pure bliss and harmony with each other and the universe. They lived in a state of enlightenment. Tantra, the art of spiritualizing sexuality, offers practical tools to transmute fear and attachment into love and universal power

Like the spring flower freeing itself from the frozen snow, Tantra is again budding, offering the Aquarian

Age an alternative—a way to reverse the negative energy on the planet, and a way to release yourself and reach transcendence. Put simply, Tantra is the total surrender, or letting go of all mental, emotional and cultural conditioning, so that universal life energy can again flow though us like a river without any effort.

It is a letting go to universal oneness...to love. When fear is removed, Tantra remains.

I. Tantra's History

The word "Tantra" has many definitions, and perhaps its real meaning has been lost to antiquity. Some scholars claim it comes from the Sanskrit or Hindi word for fabric or tapestry, meaning that it is woven into one's life. Others say that is comes from two Sanskrit words tanoti and trayati. Tanoti means to expand consciousness, and trayati means to liberate consciousness. One might then say that Tantra expands and liberates consciousness, making it the fabric of existence.

The highest possible synthesis between love and meditation, Tantra is also the connection between the third dimension and other planes of existence beyond mere materiality. While not a religious philosophy, Tantra embraces a deep spiritual understanding of life, and an ancient art of living in harmony with existence. It is a poetic science of super sexuality that dates back thousands of years, not only to India and Tibet, but to the Far East, Polynesia, and indigenous cultures of all parts of the world!, including North America's native Cherokee culture. It was used as a vehicle to achieve cosmic consciousness and union with divinity.

Tantra treats sexual energy as a loving friend, rather than something to be suppressed or talked about secretly in low tones. It does not deny sex, or consider sex a hindrance to enlightenment or Heavenly Grace. To the contrary, Tantra is the only spiritual path that says that sex is sacred, and not a sin, or something against God, whether in a marriage or not. Tantrikas are God-loving, rather than God-fearing.

There is a most beautiful word for sex in the Sanskrit language, and that is Kama, which means sex-love together, undivided and indivisible. In Tantra, sex is always loving. Almost everyone is familiar with the 7th century classic the Kama Sutra, a Tantric treatise on lovemaking. Kama is also the name of the Hindu Goddess of love. And love is what Tantra encourages—total unconditional love, including the mind, the spiritual and the body.

Tantra doesn't tell you to control or suppress your sexual urges to reach God, but rather says the opposite. It supports development of this vital energy to achieve union with Divinity. The essence of Tantra is the full expression of being—a merging with, rather than a withdrawing from. It is the ultimate yoga, which is Sanskrit for union. In Tantra, the orgasm is with the universe. You become part of the primal energy of everything. In the Kama Sutra, genital contact is but one of the many kinds of intercourse. Tantrikas learn to make love with everything, letting go of all barriers to pure bliss.

Sex becomes sacred and divine when you approach it from your heart and body, rather than your mind. It is common for Tantrikas to "drop their mind" when engaging in Tantric lovemaking. When the energy comes from a space deep within you—your essential Self—it connects you to God/Goddess/All That Is...moving you into the realm of spirit.

The body is only layers of invisible energy in form, and it

can be awakened if we let go to the sexual energy. This is the way of Tantra. It affirms the life energy within you in totality, so that those on this path find themselves whole and self-confident, with a positive panoramic view of everything.

Tantra changes one's view of relationships as well. Tantrikas are less co-dependent, jealous or neurotic. They tend to be harmonious, fun and energy-filled. In the way of Tantra, you also discover that the relationship you seek outside is already within you. You simply need to learn about and cultivate the Tantric vision, a vital, bliss-filled approach to sex, love and life in general.

II. Primal Energy

Today, many people have been exposed to the use of energy for healing, as with Chinese medicine, Reiki, Touch for Health, etc. Yet, few people, except for the Taoists, use the body's most powerful energy center—the sex center—for the achievement of divinity, immortality and enlightenment.

In Tantra, sexual energy is used as the ignition for firing the Kundalini force, the body's biological life-energy system, merging it/you with universal energy. Mystics and metaphysicians call this reaching or achieving Godhead, Nirvana, Samadhi, Mookshaor union with Divinity.

However, unlike Taoism (which actually stemmed from ancient Tantra) that says bring your energy inside for longevity, Tantra says let it go..let it all go! There is no reason to hang onto anything if eternity exists.

In Tantra, sex is used as the Cosmic union of opposites to create the polarity charge, or potential, that connects with the primordial energy from which everything in the universe arises—the totality of ALL.

On the Tantric path, we learn to use sexual energy in an extended way, not denying the physical (though nothing is really physical), but going further...deeper...higher. We dance with the electromagnetic force field of our partner, and that dance leads to Cosmic oneness. When this energy is matched and balanced correctly through a loving surrender with a partner, the sparks fly. In that moment of sexual embrace and energy exchange, a couple may achieve a Cosmic orgasm, with their essential selves exiting the body.

Those who claim to read auras can often tell if people are Tantrikas. In Tantra we learn to open ourselves to others, not only on the physical but on all levels. Yes become more prominent in our vocabulary...

The basic difference between unenlightened sex and Tantra, is that Tantra declares "the kingdom of God is within your heart." In Sanskrit it is called Pinde So Brahamande, "the physical body is the temple of God, and the body is the replica or representa! tion of the entire Cosmos."

II. 21st Century Spirituality

Contemporary society considers neurosis and deviant behavior normal, no more a problem than the common cold. Our present social and cultural structure supports separation and has created division among individuals and nations, manifesting in violence, war and in general a world without beauty and love. Western (and now even Eastern) culture uses sex for manipulation—sexy models being used to sell cars, soap and other products—while at the same time suppressing sexual expression. With sex being such a powerful force, we have created the perfect environment for neurosis, and sexual violence.

Tantra says we can celebrate life when the idea of separation, or otherness, disappears from the body and mind, allowing people to meet on all levels of consciousness—physical, vital, mental, intellectual and spiritual. In fact, Tantric partners often consider themselves "soul partners."

Tantra, the art of spiritualizing your sexuality, offers practical tools to transmute fear and attachment into love and universal power. Jealousy, possessiveness, guilt and other negative emotions that drain your life-force energy, drop away.

While most fundamentalist religions—even Eastern and Arabian philosophies—focus on the elimination of sensual pleasures, Tantra welcomes the full expression of bodily pleasure, recognizing that in the body is hidden the "bodiless," or the spiritual. The body is only layers of invisible energy in form, and it can all be awakened if we let go to the sexual energy.

The art of tantra should not be mistaken for material hedonism. Perhaps it could be called "spiritual hedonism," which says, "eat, drink and be merry, but with full awareness." Remain awake as you enter into sex before the old habits come and take over. Just remain conscious of the energy. Tantra says Yes! to sex, Yes! to love, and Yes! Yes! Yes! to unconditional love.

III. Enlightenment Now!

If you can learn to be conscious of the body and the breath, you can become conscious of the Universe.

What Buddha said can be said of Tantra, "The truth of the Universe can only be realized within the framework of the physical body."

So, while Tantra is associated with sexuality, it is essentially a merging with oneness, using the physical plane as the launch pad. We indeed create our own reality says Tantra, and this reality can be in the here and now—in the body through the Tantric orgasm. While it is possible to study Tantra for years, learning technique, meditations, and nuances, of the Tantric lifestyle, the very essence of Tantra assumes you already have all the knowledge to become enlightened immediately. DO IT NOW! Life ! wasn't meant to be a struggle.